Doctoring Together

A physician's guide to manners, duties and communication in the shared care of patients

John D. Stoeckle, Laurence J. Ronan
Linda Emanuel, Carol Ehrlich
Cynthia Cardon Hughes

Massachusetts General Hospital
Stoeckle Center for Primary Care
Primary Care Division
Harvard Medical School

This publication is made possible in part through a grant from the Pfizer Medical Humanities Initiative, along with support from Partners HealthCare Systems and Massachusetts General Hospital.

This publication is made possible in part through a grant from the Pfizer Medical Humanities Initiative, along with support from Partners HealthCare Systems and Massachusetts General Hospital.

Printed in the United States of America

Massachusetts General Hospital
15 Parkman St., WAC 620
Boston, MA 02114

Library of Congress Cataloging-in-Publication Data

Doctoring Together

1. Doctor-Doctor relationships 2. Doctor-Nurse relationships
I. Stoeckle JD, Ronan LJ, Emanuel LL, Ehrlich CH, Hughes CC
II. Title [DNLM: 1. Shared Care of Patients 4. Communication among health care professionals]

ISBN 0-9720462-0-8

Contents

is, therefore, part of our professionalism. In that way, this manual is an important contribution to the literature of professionalism.

The physicians at Partners have expressed their professionalism by agreeing on a set of "Principles of Patient Care." These were developed by a representative group of Partners physicians, modified after a review by several hundred more, and ultimately ratified by all the physician groups, representing 11 institutions and nearly 7000 physicians.

These "Principles," included in the appendix, are notable in how many of them deal with aspects of the physician to physician communication discussed in this manual.

The MGH has a long tradition of leadership in professional issues. This manual fits well into the body of work by pre-eminent physicians, such as Holmes, Cabot, Shattuck, Means, Bauer, Knowles, and others. It also fits well with the professional aspirations of the physicians within Partners HealthCare System and of practicing physicians everywhere.

G.E. Thibault, M.D.
Vice President of Clinical Affairs
Partners HealthCare Systems, Inc.
Professor of Medicine
Harvard Medical School

Introduction

"You didn't know I was admitted!"

"Doctor Jones didn't send you a report on what he did?"

"Doctor Good said I didn't need all those tests and should have come sooner."

"I like coming here because I know that all you doctors will get together to find out what's wrong with me."

**Patients on doctors,
circa 1997**

They had found here certain ethical and intellectual standards taken as a matter of course. I mean, a wise man's honest confession of ignorance, the absence of suspicion, secrecy, and backbiting, the rule of fairness to others, the habitual thoroughness of examination, record, and subsequent study, the habitual courtesy under conditions which tempt us to a bold and mechanical type of "intercourse..."

Richard C. Cabot, Ether Day Address, 1919[1]

guide doctors' behavior toward others who work in health care, will assist all practitioners who value excellence.

CHAPTER I

Doctoring Together

We are all brothers and sisters…

Hippocrates

To cure sometimes, to relieve often, to comfort always.

Folk saying
15th century or earlier

To prevent disease, to relieve suffering,
and to heal the sickness, this is our work.

Sir William Osler[16]

Introduction

Doctoring together means doing well by patients by doing good by one another. And doing good by one another means providing mutual support, from showing interest in the clinical work and careers of other physicians to mentoring physicians-in-training and sharing the care of a patient with colleagues. In doctoring together today, the common shared tasks of care include:[17, 18]

- **Accurate diagnosis and effective treatment** (indeed, cost-effective treatment) of the patient's medical-psychological illness
- **Communication of information** to the patient and family about illness, its diagnosis, treatment, prevention, and prognosis
- **Personal support** of patients of all backgrounds, in all stages of illness, with shared decision-making in their diagnosis and treatment
- **Optimal maintenance and rehabilitation** of the chronically disabled
- **Prevention**, when possible, of the patient's disease and disablements through risk assessment, early disease diagnosis, health education, and preventive treatment

How the Organization of Medical Care Has Changed Doctor-Doctor Relationships

As we grow in size and numbers will we be able to keep the Jackson-Warren spirit? Or as we develop into a huge and diversified industry shall we become as mechanical and soulless as a factory?

— **Richard C. Cabot, Ether Day Address, 1919**[1]

...The present crux in which the medical profession finds itself, overmanned, overspecialized, like other necessities of life poorly distributed, an expensive luxury for those of modest means and subject of investigation...unless we promptly do something to alter our spots, to cast off our long-conditioned reflexes, and put ourselves on a modern chain store business.

— **Harvey Cushing, The Medical Career, 1933**[19]

Before providing advice on "doctoring together," the authors of this manual feel compelled to comment on how the changing organization of medical practice and the market culture of care redefine relationships among us — sometimes making work together more difficult, and, sometimes, easier. In brief, care today has become more divided, corporate, competitive, bigger, managed, costly, communicated, standardized, and, we hope, shared. These changes create new conditions for our professional relationships in the care of patients. What follows are nine truths about care today:

Care Is Divided Practice specializes and grows more technical. Professional relationships, in turn, divide among themselves and sometimes fragment altogether. As a result, specialists often conduct care with little collaboration or coordination,[20] dispersing patients among one another without acknowledgment of the need for, or communication with, a primary care practitioner (PCP). This pattern of specialist-to-specialist care, where the patient seeks care and receives referrals from multiple specialists, nowadays goes by the term "split care."

Care Is Corporate The corporate organization of practice (hospitals and HMOs) and the regulations of payers and health care plans (managed care and insurers) often specify which doctors a patient may consult and where this consultation may take place. Thus, the insurer — rather than the doctor — "owns" the patient. Indeed, the insurer may even "own" the MD.[21, 22]

The network of approved colleagues and conditions for consultation referral, for the shared care of patients between practitioners, has become less restrictive. Nonetheless, not only does the insurer control the process, but the practitioner's own financial incentive also plays a role.[23] Despite the preferences and needs of practitioner and patient, the previous traditional, informal, reciprocal consultative exchange by the doctor among his/her choices of colleagues no longer fuels practice. In addition, the published guidelines of specialty groups of MDs drive decision- making. Teams within an organization reach a consensus (e.g., those pain, breast, and stroke "centers") about a patient; no longer does a doctor always consult with whomever he or she chooses.

Care Is Competitive While care of patients in group practices has boundaries, a market culture of care gives patients self-referral access to physicians, groups, and institutions — an abundance of choices that may lead patients to engage and exit professional relationships quickly. At the same time, the annual re-enrollment provisions of insurance plans, and changing contracts between employers and insurers for the least expensive plan, also disconnect patients from their PCPs and from their physicians' consulting colleagues. Patients then lose choice. And when patients seek consultations on their own, their selected practitioners may have no tradition, incentive, or demand to communicate with colleagues who have been providing the patients' continuing care.

Similarly, consulting specialists may no longer hold the old ethos of transmitting knowledge and skill (and the patient) back to the generalist. Market competition drives the modem ethos of attracting more "customers" or "clientele." Indeed, on one hand, outcome measures play a significant role in the science and politics of specialist versus generalist competition today. Some studies demonstrate a lower mortality with AIDS and heart disease patients, for example, when specialists rather than PCPs care for patients.[24] Studies of other conditions, such as hypertension, show no outcome differences.[25] So far, no outcomes studies analyze the possible greater benefit if specialists and PCPs co-manage patients.

Yet some specialty societies (arthritis, for example) jointly with primary care practitioners define the decision-trees for patients' diagnosis and treatment.[26] Such guidelines should bring about better, appropriate co-management of patients.

Overall, the various market choices appear to offer patients cheaper premiums and more choices of practitioners. Yet the options may, in fact, be fewer — and for doctors, too. Patients who contract with new practice plans may lack, at least temporarily, connecting consultations that might improve the doctor-doctor coordination of their care.

Care Is Bigger, Diversified Practice organizations have grown so large and diversified that professional contacts among practitioners are not only more numerous, but often far less personal, informal, long-term, or face-to-face. Our profession has 800,000 MDs — up 28 percent since 1980 — with over 60 percent in some form of group practice. More and more, doctors exchange information with one another by phone calls, institutional mail, record notes, and, sometimes, even "telemedicine."[27] Electronic mail with its speed and directness may either improve practitioner exchange[28] or, ironically, increase impersonal professional connections, with fewer face-to-face meetings and hallway-corridor conversations.

In teaching institutions, weak relationships may become a way of life because the staff-in-training is not only large but transient in their institutional lives. Residencies, which last three to six years, consist of two- to three-month training rotations in multiple hospital services. Moreover, no longer do small all-male clubs rule our increasingly large practice organizations. Whether hospital networks, HMOs, groups, or PPOs, practice plans operate with "physician networks" in which diversity — by age, gender, race, ethnicity, national origins, and training abroad — occurs as a matter of course.[29]

Care Is Managed By "doctoring," practitioners often speak of managing patients' care and treatment — ancient roles of the profession. But management of another kind, namely managing doctors, also dominates doctor-doctor relationships today. Physician managers work inside practices as well as outside for insurers and managed care firms.

Outside of practices, managers monitor doctors' decisions on the use of tests, procedures, and treatments for approved insurance coverage with increasing scrutiny. Inside practices, management programs such as TQM (Total Quality Management) and CQI (Continuous Quality Improvement) strive to improve quality of care, not only its efficiency (though it should be acknowledged that today efficiency is the chief motivation).[30] In both settings, these physician manager-doctor relationships reflect a corporate model of middle management — one that struggles to move an hierarchical management culture to a collaborative one.[31]

In some instances, for example, the physician manager relates with staff doctors as one of their group, stimulating collaborative work and developing group consensus on "pathways of care" and clinical practices. In other instances, the physician manager supervises the individual practitioner or group. A manager may be placed in this role by the practice or the insurance plan.

A manager's focus on the mistakes of an individual physician or group of physicians (diagnoses, case management, treatment, and productivity) can produce a potentially critical, authoritative exchange that, too often, shames the practitioner or staff. Educated in the belief that professionalism equals accountability, doctors want to set the standards of medical work at the point of patient care — not to have standards set above that care or exterior to it by managers.[32]

Care Is Communicated In practice organizations, technologies such as electronic mail, fax, computers and other equipment ease and even change professional communication.[33, 34] They can also be used to monitor staff decisions. To improve doctor- doctor exchanges, institutions must invest in these communication technologies in optimal ways. Too often, however, technical training and support break down, resulting in failure to protect such rights as the confidentiality of the patient's record.

Care Is Standardized Today's corporate practice requires more doctoring together, not only for the needs of the individual patient but also for the needs of the practice population. Many doctors believe that group decisions on standards of care for all practitioners, not only for physicians but other health professions, e.g., nursing, improve treatment.[35]

First, group practice decisions on the organizational process of care may improve care for all persons in a practice population, enhancing, in turn, the personal care of the individual patient.

Second, group practice decisions on the appropriate treatment and use of resources, namely new practice guidelines for practice populations, may influence, in turn, the practitioner's personal care. In both situations, these group decisions among members of the profession's specialties are a kind of doctoring together that is focused on practice populations, not the individual patient.[36] Negotiating these decisions, of course, may be difficult, complicated by professional self-interest, power, status, and distrust. Some of the often-conflicted, often-ignored boundary and jurisdictional issues for group decisions by specialists and generalists include the following:

- **Appropriate use of medical technologies** in diagnosis and treatment
- **Design of effective clinical care processes** for diagnosis, treatment, and rehabilitation
- **Priority in therapeutic responsibility and professional fees** in the co-management of patients
- **Costs of technical testing** and charges for such services
- **Use of new therapies** (e.g., proscar by generalist versus specialist)
- **Pay of professional staff** and the need for differentials, if any, between specialists and generalists.

Care Is Costly The costs of care influence doctor-doctor relations today, yesterday and forever more. At the moment, however, the "bottom line" is a paramount concern. Institutions and professionals often "go where the money is," though not so easily as insurers and others restrict resources for health care. Wishing to control costs, policy experts strive to limit the overproduction (supply) of physicians and the costs physicians generate. Meanwhile the public, managers, and practitioners on their own have begun to define appropriate technology use that may limit demand. Indeed, group practices with more restricted resources and larger numbers of physicians will force reconsideration of the design, organization, and payment of clinical care.

The much higher reward for specialist compared with generalist physician contributes to the costs of professional services, the attraction of specialist careers, and professional disharmony over practice rewards.[37] Specialists, generalists and non-physician health workers need a more open consensus on tasks and rewards.

Practitioners themselves must work with institutional managers and physician managers to reduce costs, improve treatments and design decision-making processes on medical work and pay that make sense.

Care Is Shared Fortunately, physicians today are less hierarchical in professional relationships, not only with each other but also with nurses, social workers, and other health care practitioners. Specialization and technology that demand teamwork propel these changes, as do the social press for more equality in and among the professions and the development of part-time shared practices.

Some physicians, no longer full-time in any one practice, easily exchange patients, records, and the coverage of co-practitioners and nursing colleagues. These modern generalist physicians provide an historical example of shared care transforming interprofessional relations. As chronic care rather than acute illness dominates practice and moves outside the hospital to group practices, the generalist no longer dwells in a vertical relationship with the specialist. Some reflections on the past and present relationship of PCP and specialist show the significance of this change.

A Brief History of Medical Practice

At one time general practitioners or "GPs" occupied the bottom of a three-tiered organizational hierarchy. After providing community-based services (primary care), GPs might move some patients on and up to specialists (secondary care), and to hospitals (tertiary care) for complex decisions on diagnosis and treatment — decisions often carried out without their participation. The GP's clinical administrative care provided the functions of initial access, continuity, and coordination.[38] Many physicians, particularly specialists, viewed the GP's work as general care of ordinary bodily complaints —"sniffles and sneezes," "gas and indigestion," "aches and pains," "nerves and worries."

By contrast, today's modern generalist physicians (now specialists, too, as pediatricians, internists, and family practitioners), play a central position on a horizontal field of exchange with subspecialists outside the hospital. Over the last three decades, hospital-based diagnostic treatment technologies have been decentralized to ambulatory sites that, in turn, have moved much hospital medicine into out-patient practices where the generalist uses nearly the same high-tech testing as the specialist.[39]

More and more, generalists work in an exchange with specialists in group practices. The scope of the management of acute and chronic illness is also broader, carried out in group practices by both generalists and sub-specialists. Indeed, primary care practitioners (PCPs) today regularly engage in illness management of the patient's several co-morbid disorders, some complex as well as ordinary, some requiring the subspecialist's opinion, diagnostic technique, and treatment (Fig. 1).

As a result of the public's search for early diagnosis, treatment, and prevention by consulting the PCP, decision-making around these tasks is now shared through interprofessional and patient interaction. Modern medicine has transformed the old hierarchical arrangements. No longer does the PCP refer patients "upward" to specialists who separately pursue diagnosis and treatment.

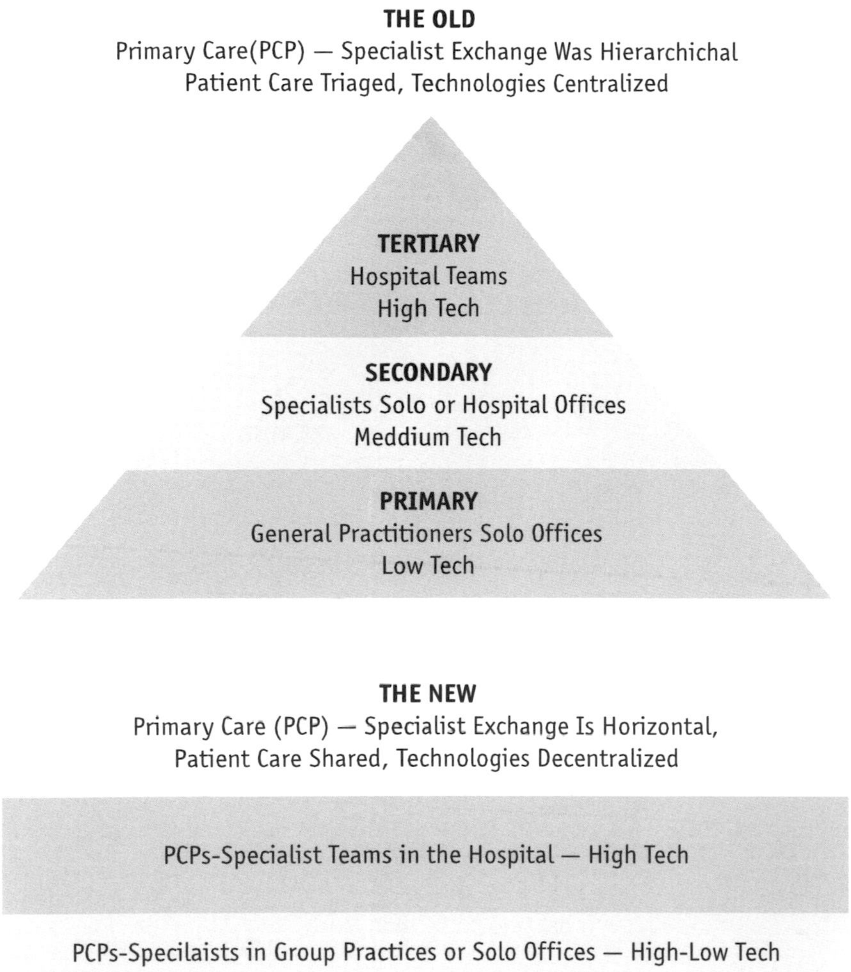

THE OLD

Primary Care(PCP) — Specialist Exchange Was Hierarchichal
Patient Care Triaged, Technologies Centralized

TERTIARY
Hospital Teams
High Tech

SECONDARY
Specialists Solo or Hospital Offices
Meddium Tech

PRIMARY
General Practitioners Solo Offices
Low Tech

THE NEW

Primary Care (PCP) — Specialist Exchange Is Horizontal,
Patient Care Shared, Technologies Decentralized

PCPs-Specialist Teams in the Hospital — High Tech

PCPs-Specilaists in Group Practices or Solo Offices — High-Low Tech

Figure 1 Professional Relationships, Old and New

Medical Practice Today

"The day of the general practitioner is passing...but the day of the isolated specialist has also begun to pass."

E.A. Codman, A Study in Hospital Efficiency, 1916[40]

It is well-known that organizational changes in and around medical practice often make doctors more accountable to interest groups outside the profession than to each other. Professional solidarity in the common work of patient care thus diminishes. These changes significantly influence doctor-doctor relationships, depending on the attitude and values of the individual practitioner, his/her specialty group, and the clinic in which subspecialists often provide general care along with specialty care. Primary care physicians may have one view, subspecialists another, while practice administrators and non-physician health practitioners, still others.

That the central, equal, no longer subordinate position of the PCP in collaboration with subspecialists is a given, reflects the perspective of the authors — all primary care practitioners. (Although subspecialists outnumber generalists 70 percent to 30 percent, many professionals propose returning to an older balance of a 50-50 "health manpower" mix.) Unlike the separation of subspecialists and generalists in Codman's day, both today have access to modern diagnostic technology. The PCP not only provides care but also co-manages illness along with patients and subspecialists; thus the primary care practitioner plays an essential role in a specialized profession — not an obsolete one as some suggest. In this modern specialist-generalist mix, better doctor-doctor communication matters for patient care.

A desire to improve the effectiveness and civility of interprofessional relationships that are no longer hierarchical also motivates this manual's authors. And, finally, the authors want to view the market reorganization of medical practice with optimism and suggest constructive changes. These tasks demand renewed attention to our professionalism and our communication with each other in the shared care of patients.

The advice and illustrated doctor-doctor relations which follow stem from the practice experiences of the authors at the Massachusetts General Hospital (its clinics, group practices and health centers), even though illustrations might just as easily be used from community-based colleagues who report similar experiences. Regardless, these accounts bear on our modern and traditional doctor-doctor connections and communication. Four professional relationship themes are addressed: Doctor-Doctor, Doctor-Resident, Doctor-Student teaching, and Doctor-Nurse.

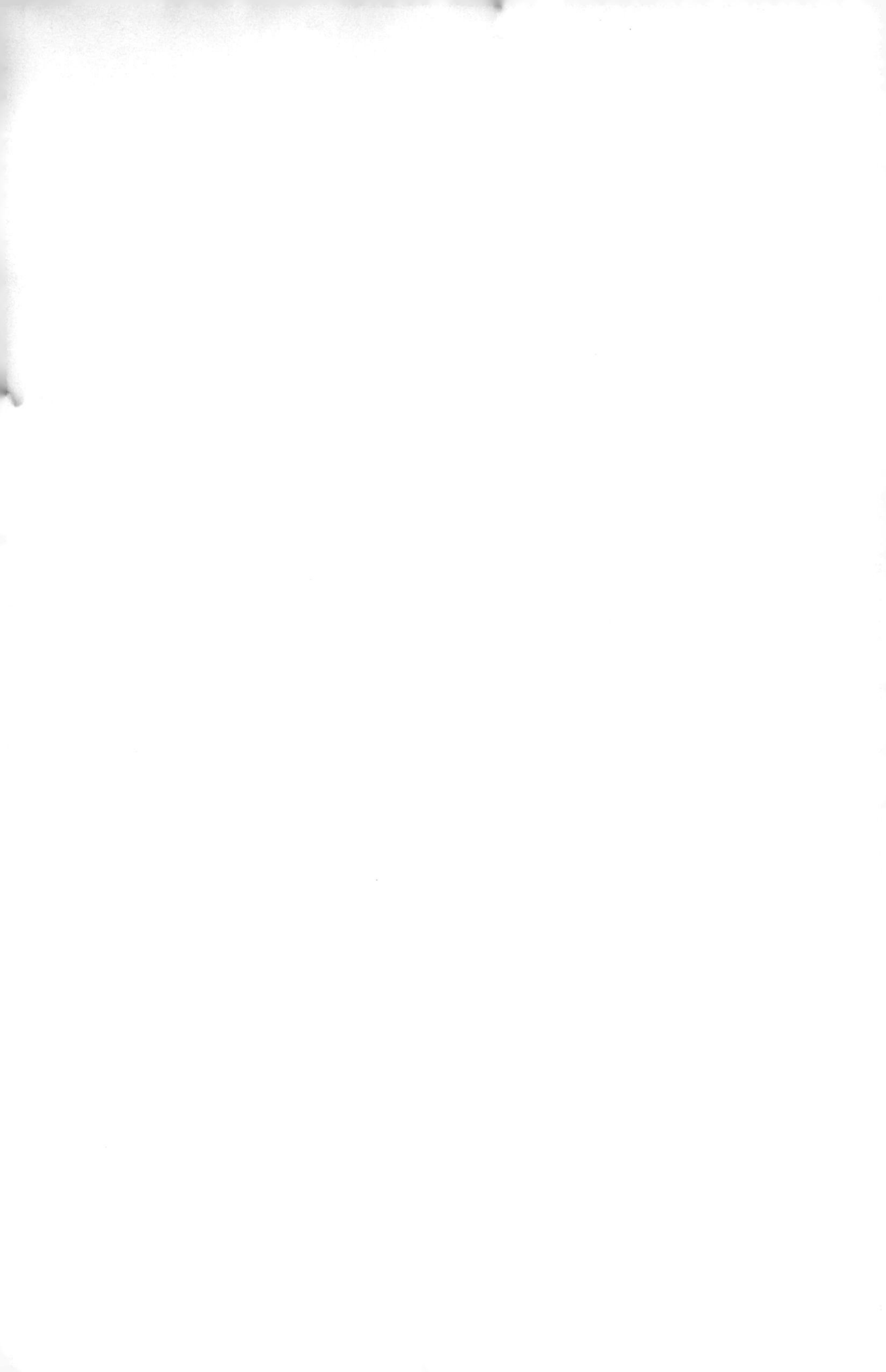

Doctor-Doctor Relationships

"Miss Manners does not want people to act naturally; she wants them to act civilly."

A. Hulburt
Why Manners Matter, 1982[41]

"By their intercourse with each other, physicians will best consult and secure their own self-respect and consideration from society in general, by a universal courtesy and high-minded conduct towards their professional brethren."

AMA Medical Ethics, June 5, 1947[42]

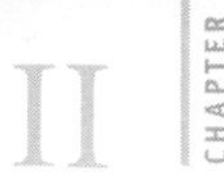

On Institutional Manners

Despite an awareness of professional manners, doctors easily forget that the patient relates to a variety of health care professionals both inside and outside the hospital: the PCP, other physicians, nurses, home-health aides, physical therapists and others. And, of course, the patient may possess an informal network of caretakers, such as his/her family and friends. Cooperative and cordial relationships among the patient's practitioners make for the patient's welfare. In the service of that welfare, here are some everyday manners for the hospital and office practice.[43]

Notification of Admission/Discharge

Upon admitting a patient to the hospital from the emergency ward or staff offices inside or outside the hospital, practitioners should notify the patient's PCP (whether on or off the hospital staff) and later provide discharge plans in time for follow-up visits (see example on facing page). Similarly, surgical and specialty colleagues should notify the PCP about the admission/discharge of any patients they admit.

Such courtesy notifications, carried out independently of seeking a formal consultation with the PCP to discuss patient care, serve both patients and doctors. For patients, the notification may result in a personal visit by the PCP that provides a reassuring doctor-patient connection. For the PCP, the visit may inform him/her about the patient's illness and treatments, maintaining, in turn, solidarity among professionals working together. Such notification benefits the patient, the PCP, and the staff. Incidentally, hospital staff should make these admission/discharge notifications not only by telephone, but also by letter and hospital discharge summary.

Here's one doctor's brief, factual letter to another doctor.

Example of an Admission Notification

Dear William,

A note to let you know that your patient Mrs. X has been scheduled for admission for her TKR on 8/15/92.

Sincerely, Dr. P.K.

Result: The PCP saw the patient during her recovery and got a first-hand account of her experience.

Bottom Line: An admission notification a) serves the patient, and b) serves good doctor-doctor relationships.

Here's how doctors let down a patient and a PCP.

A Failure to Provide Discharge Information

A 48-year-old man was seen in the emergency room on self-referral early in the morning for atypical chest pain. Though he had multiple cardiac risk factors, the patient's history, examination, and laboratory data, including a resting EKG when in pain, were unconvincing. An exercise stress test was arranged from the emergency room two days later, which was markedly positive. The record documented the PCP, but the patient was discharged without the PCP's knowledge. When the patient appeared in the PCP's office for a follow-up visit, he was angry that his care and test results were unknown.

Result: The PCP quickly pursued and reviewed the findings, and then excused the ER staff's oversight without reviewing the care process with that staff.

Bottom Line: Prevention means not only identifying the PCP or specialist MD at each step of the care process, including testing, but also going over lapses in communication between and among doctors.

Here's how a patient received unnecessary tests in the hospital.

A Misuse of an Admission Notification

A 70-year-old patient with advanced cancer was admitted for chemotherapy, managed by the oncologist. The PCP was notified as a courtesy, but used the occasion of being notified to undertake an exam and tests that were neither needed nor discussed.

Result: The behavior of the PCP was deemed inappropriate by the consulting oncologist, but the oncologist did not discuss the matter with the PCP.

Bottom Line: An admission notification from one doctor to another is a reality of shared care that should never be abused. The PCP should have discussed his/her wish with the oncologist to do an exam and tests of the patient; the two doctors should have then made a decision together that best served the patient's interests.

Documenting the PCP Relationship

The patient's medical record should document that he/she has a PCP (a continuing professional source of medical care in the community, or on the hospital's staff, or in an affiliated practice), and should serve as an institutional reminder of the need to communicate information when staff admit, transfer, or discharge a patient. That documentation can be made at several sites:

In the Patient's Hospital Record The admission medical history should contain the name, address, and telephone number of the patient's PCP, as in Fig. 4. This recording practice should also list the resident physician-in-training as the PCP, if he/she provides primary care to the patient in any of the ambulatory practices of the institution — its clinics, health centers, teaching group practices or private offices. Because some patients are confused upon admission and cannot identify their PCP, staff may need to elicit the information from family members or friends.

THE GENERAL HOSPITAL

UNIT: 018-73-41
NAME: Frances Jones
ADDRESS: 17 Court St., Woburn,MA 01880
DATE: 2/15/96

ADMISSION NOTE
PC Physician: Dr. W. A.Smith,220 Hanover, Boston,MA
Tel: 617-227-4128

HISTORY
Mrs. Frances Jones is a 70-year-old retired secretary admitted because of increasing shortness of breath and intermittent chest pain in the past 4 days....

Figure 4 The Patient's Recorded History

In the Hospital and EW Admission Sheets Besides the clinical recording of the patient's PCP in the medical history, staff should also record this information on admission sheets (Fig. 5) to the EW and the hospital.

THE GENERAL HOSPITAL

Admit Date: 10/1/82	**Admit Time:** 10:00 AM
Service: Med	**Room/Bed:** 444
Unit: 018-73-41	**Sex:** F
Soc Sec: 315-46-7700	**Mar St.:** M
DOB: 9-10-22	**Age:** 70

Patient Name: Jones, Frances A.
Address: 17 Court St., Woburn, MA 01880

Contact: Jones, William A.
Relation: H
Home Tel.: 781-721-7760
City/State: Woburn, MA 01880

Admitting Physician: James Burke
Attending Physician: William A. Smith
Primary Care Physician: William A. Smith

Figure 5 The Admission Sheet

Fig. 6 shows documentation of the PCP and other consultants in the hospital discharge summary.

THE GENERAL HOSPITAL

NAME: Frances Jones **UNIT:** 018-73-41
ADMITTED: 10/1/92 **DISCHARGED:** 10/7/92
DIAGNOSES:...
HISTORY:...
PHYSICAL:...
HOSPITAL COURSE:...
DISCHARGE MEDICATIONS: John R. Rouse, M.D.
cc: William A. Smith, M.D., PCP
cc: Richard Jones, M.D

Figure 6 The Patient's Discharge Summary

THE GENERAL HOSPITAL

018-73-41

JONES, FRANCES A.
17 COURT STREET
WOBURN, MA 01880

Mass HMO Blue
PCP: Dr. William Smith

Figure 7 The Patient's Identification Card

In the Office, Outpatient or Ambulatory Practice Record

The patient's identification card should label the PCP name on each stamped record sheet (Fig. 7). In the case of outpatient records, many do not regularly document the PCP. Nor do the records of PCPs often document the consultants to patients. Such lack of documentation harms professional communication in group practice. Very likely, managed care will demand documentation through administrative rules similar to those that require coordination of consultation/ referrals through PCPs, while group practice electronic records will contain the documentation of all staff.

Besides the identification carried on the patient's card, the office write-up of the consultation (Fig. 8) can also carry information about the PCP.

Office Notes: JAS, #53964, Visit, January 10, 1993
Attending Physician: Dr. D. H. James.
Referring Physician: Dr. W. A. Smith, 220 Hanover Street, Boston, MA 02113.

JAS is seen in follow-up after coronary bypass surgery. He is already doing a considerable amount of physical activity and has lost weight. His lipids appear acceptable. He is on digoxin, aspirin, and his asthma inhalers. He is doing breathing exercises to improve his lung expansion. He looks fit and is asymptomatic. An echocardiogram performed today continues to show basal akinesis.

His overall ventricular function is good, however, and his ejection fraction is probably around 55 percent. He continues to have considerable ectopic activity noted on his echo. This had been reviewed prior to discharge, and an EP study was performed which led to the conclusion that he did not need antiarrhythmic therapy. I did not examine him today. I only discussed the issues with him. Plan: (1) Discontinue digoxin; (2) Continue aspirin, diet, exercise, and weight loss as he is doing; and (3) 1 would like to have him undergo a regular exercise test before he leaves for his vacation. I will arrange for that and send a copy of the results to his primary care physician, Dr. Smith. After that, I will be returning him to Dr. Smith's care.

s/ Douglas H. James, M.D.

cc: W. A. Smith, M.D.

Figure 8 Office Documentation as Follow-Up Letter

Unfortunately, the PCP is not systematically recorded in the hospital record, admission sheet, discharge summary, office note, or on the identification card and office documentation — despite the fact that this information may contribute to patient care. Nor does the PCP regularly receive information from other caregivers, though with competitive procedures, consultant replies are vastly more common and prompt than ever before.

The following instance, as well as surveys of consultation referrals, makes this point. In this case, a university hospital shuts out a PCP, and lets a patient down.

Missing Documentation, Missing Communication

A 72-year-old woman is admitted by the ward resident team for a lung mass that on evaluation is an adenocarcinoma. Her primary care physician of twenty years is a community doctor without admitting privileges at the university hospital. Nowhere in the chart is the doctor's name noted in the patient's history though the doctor is referred to as the patient's "LMD." No call is sent from the resident team inquiring about prior evaluation, nor on discharge are current evaluation or management plans transmitted. As a consequence, the PCP, who later provides terminal care, is initially embarrassed because of being uninformed when the patient returns to the office for follow-up.

Result: No feedback was given the institution or staff by the PCP who lacked staff connections.

Bottom Line: Prevention means education of staff to recognize the connection of patients to colleagues (even if not staff), and common work of care in and outside the hospital.

On Professional Exchange Forms of Address

Senior staff should discourage labeling the Primary Care Physician as LMD (Local Medical Doctor), because of its historical pejorative status and the fact that the PCP is not necessarily local. Historically,

"LMD" served as the hospital staff's label for the patient's community practitioner — an anonymous colleague often excluded from hospital staff membership, a physician whose name students, residents, and consultants rarely note in recording the patient's medical history. Today, practitioners should encourage the term "PCP" for its descriptive accuracy of the role of primary care physicians.

First Names If "LMD" is out, so is formal address between doctors — for the most part. First names are in. Away from the bedside and office rounds with patients, juniors should feel comfortable being on a first-name basis with seniors. Yet all physicians, senior and junior staff alike, should well understand appropriate behavior among staff. Being on a first-name basis no longer indicates familiarity, but rather equality.

Introductions Informality aside, introductions still serve an important and necessary function among the staff. Name tags do not substitute for preemptive personal introductions of oneself and one's role: "I'm doctor V" or "I'm Jane X, the cardiac fellow." Such spontaneous introductions of ourselves as newcomers to each other on hospital wards, rounds, practices, consultations, and conferences should prevent confusion, embarrassment, and quizzes from the staff as to "Who are you?"

Telephone Calls, Calling and Answering

Phoning staff and other colleagues is an important means of interprofessional communication over and beyond the formality of written exchanges. Occasions for calling include:

- **Hospital admission**
- **Hospital discharge**
- **Major crisis events** in hospital
- **Operative findings and conditions**

- **Initiation of consultation referrals**
- **Patient death**

Staff sometimes delay making phone calls because a death, acute deterioration or other crisis occurs after the attending physician's working hours. Such delay is not acceptable.

Practitioners should answer phone calls or pages from physician-colleagues, even if the calls may interrupt office consultations with patients. If offered an "excuse me," patients invariably accept such interruptions on behalf of another patient's care.

Communication in Writing

Staff should report to the PCP and referring colleagues in writing any hospitalizations, emergency ward and walk-in-service visits, and office consultation-referrals. Thanking colleagues for consultation referrals may appear a bit old-fashioned, or even seem disingenuous when that patient is burdensome and difficult. Yet the spirit of thanking one's colleague, and thereby endorsing the exchange, is essential professionalism (see Fig. 9).

> Dr. William Smith
> 220 Hanover Street
> Boston, MA 02113
>
> Dear Dr. Smith:
>
> Just a note in follow-up of the discharge summary sent on Mr. John Hunter. His TURP on 2/10/99 was without complications. He was seen 3/1/99, and was without his usual nocturia, which was resolving. He will be returning to you for continuing care. Thank you for the consultation and referral.
>
> John Jones, M.D.

Figure 9 Thank You Letter for Consultation Referral

On Consulting Together

Consultations should be promoted, in difficult or protracted cases, as they give rise to confidence, energy, and more enlarged views in practice. On such occasions no rivalship or jealousy should be indulged. Candor, probity, and all due respect should be exercised towards the physician or surgeon first engaged; and as he may be presumed to be best acquainted with the patient and his family, he should deliver all the medical directions agreed upon….

T. Percival, Medical Ethics, 1803[44]

Practitioners in Great Britain more than the United States have researched and written on a variety of themes about consultations: (1) how many; (2) who gets them; (3) the form, content and timing of the information exchanged by the PCP and consultant; (4) the satisfactions of PCPs and consultants; and (5) advice in improving their communications and relationships.

In brief, the literature indicates that consultations vary from 1.5 to 10% of medical visits and are usually split between surgical and medical subspecialists. Older doctors rather than younger doctors[45-47] initiate consultations more often,[48-50] transmitting their requests by letter and sometimes by phone. Unfortunately, the consultative information exchanged often does not meet the needs of the consultant or the PCP.[51-53]

Other Uses of Consultations

Consultations have varied uses; some that physicians rarely address explicitly include the following:

- **Testing procedures,** e.g., colonoscopy, essential for accurate diagnosis and treatment
- **Confirmatory opinions of specialists** that reassure the practitioner (or the patient), endorsing that the care provided is comprehensive and accurate

- **Transfer or co-management** of one medical problem among several co-morbid conditions, deciding who is going to manage and who is going to charge
- **Specific consultant instruction** to PCPs to enable them to carry out management
- **Accommodation to patient's or family's request** for specialist opinion[54, 55]
- **Splitting care to consultants** to avoid the burden of solo management of difficult patients or simply to meet the demands of a large case load of patients
- **Medical-legal concerns** with the hope that the consultants will sanction the practitioner's care and support it if legally challenged by a malpractice suit
- **Providing additional visits** for the needs of the patient for attention and reassurance
- **Teaching,** letting other staff and trainees see unusual disorders of patients, even when recognized and appropriately managed
- **Learning,** getting more information from consultants about diagnosis and treatment

Such uses (and there may be others) of consultations may need to be made explicit among colleagues. Too often, unfortunately, conflict rather than cooperation marks consultations due to differing expectations among PCPs, patients, and specialists. Consultation requests are, at minimum, a two-way exchange. Being open and explicit about one's request can be a difficult communication style for practitioners; it needs encouragement by and a supportive response from consultants.

Specialist Response to Consultation

Specialists can neglect to support the PCP by taking over all the patient's care or by not encouraging and/or directing the patient to maintain check ups with the PCP. Emmanuel and Richter described the PCP-consultant model as a deliberative[56] one that recognizes that the consultant has communicative responsibilities not only to the referring MD, but also to the patient. Such communication focuses expectations and reduces conflict, these writers said.

This modern view of consultations contrasts to the historical admonition of Percival that specialists communicate only to the referring MD, not the patient. Most importantly, however, consultant communication with patients needs to be accompanied by the consultant's discussion, shared decision-making and co-management with the PCP.

PCP Requests for Consultation, Written and Oral

Written communications to consultants are an important duty of PCPs when seeking opinions and interventions from specialist colleagues, and from the staff of hospital services such as the EW, radiology, and testing units. Computer-based records should facilitate this communication. Sent along with a note of specific consultation request, records should transmit needed information and give the clinical details of the patient's illness.

Patients can carry these records and notes or physicians can send these items in advance. Patients with complicated conditions will require more personal communication between the PCP and consultant, such as a face-to-face meeting or phone contact. Without a written request and information transmittal, a referral consultation from the PCP to specialist is not appropriate.

In consultations on hospitalized patients, the record should indicate what specifically is requested of the consultant and by whom. Consultant requests on the order sheet alone are insufficient. A record notation is also important (Fig. 10).

```
CONSULT: Dr. Richard Lima

Would appreciate your opinion of
patient's persistent abdominal pain.
Would colonoscopy be indicated given our
studies to date?

Janet MacDonald, M.D.
```

Figure 10 Record Consultation Request

PCP Communication with Consultants

PCP communications to consultants should not be made through off-hand comments to patients: "Call Dr. 'X' for an appointment and see what he says." Instead, PCPs should pose specific questions and requests to consultants about diagnostic and treatment options (Figs. 11, 12).

> Dear Colleague:
>
> I hope you will review our care and treatment of Mrs. Jones' recent arthritis flare. Her studies are enclosed…

Figure 11 Written Request for Consultant Approval

> Dear Colleague:
>
> Patient and I would appreciate your opinion of her chronic GI distress…

Figure 12 Written Request on Patient's Behalf for Consultant Approval

Information transmittal by the PCP is also key, providing the consultant with a report of the medical work-up. Diagnostic studies nowadays are complex, even outside the hospital. The PCP no longer refers only after the history and physical, but also after imaging studies and special diagnostic lab tests that need to be exchanged with consultants in a spirit of shared decision-making and co-management.

Consultation for Testing

Referring patients for tests — radiologic, vascular, neurologic studies, etc. — requires the communication of clinical information. Such information is important for clinical staff who interpret tests. Equally important is that the PCP participate in a personal review of the findings; this procedure provides the primary care physician with a better understanding of the results and an opportunity to obtain advice on appropriate additional testing.

Consultation Responses between Consultant and PCP

The consultant should address the PCP's request for advice and relay any pertinent issues related to the patient's illness. However, consultants' gratuitous recommendations for other consultations, e.g., "Patient needs neurologic or endocrine workup" are inappropriate asides. Even if the patient needs additional consultations, the specialist should first ask the PCP about ongoing diagnostic treatment plans.

Cliches about the notoriously bad handwriting of doctors aside, appropriate communication requires that the content of any note be legible to others caring for the patient. If the signature of the consultant and the consultant's opinion is illegible, the addition of her/his name in printed letters below the signature will facilitate making a personal contact for collaborative exchange on the patient's care.

Upon completing a review of the patient, the consultant should refer the patient back to the PCP. If the consultant observes new clinical issues that may need exploration, he/she should discuss those issues with the referring PCP. Together, the consultant and the PCP can decide how to co-manage the patient — whether to contact other physicians or to request additional testing (see example below).

Failure to maintain such interprofessional exchanges may lead to a "daisy chain" of consultant-to-consultant referrals — consultant A to consultant B to consultant C — and the performance of questionable procedures (as shown on next page). Coordination with the PCP by phone or letter is essential for the needs of the patient. While managed care requires that the PCP direct all consultations as a matter of policy, such coordination should be a professional standard and not an administrative rule.

Coordinated Care: Primary Care Physician to Consultant 1 to Consultant 2 (Report of Consultant 2)

The patient of Dr. W. Smith (PCP) is a 76-year-old, white female with chronic lymphocytic lymphoma with symptomatic right axillary mass. (Patient referred to consultant-1, Dr. J. Jones (oncology). After biopsy established diagnosis, telephone agreement was made to recommend radiation, and patient was referred to Dr. Ling (radiation therapy).

Treatment Accomplished: *From 2/8/93 to 3/4/93 the patient was treated in 2.0 Gy fractions over a period of 24 days. Using AP/PA parallel opposed ports measuring 19 x 13.5 cm. the patient was treated to a total dose of 3600 cGy.*

Treatment Tolerance: *The patient tolerated the treatment well with no side effects from the radiation whatsoever. She did develop a rash from her arthritis pain medications, which was handled by her primary care physician, Dr. W. Smith.*

Disposition: *The recommendations are for the patient to follow up with Dr. Jones (oncology) and Dr. Smith (PCP). Dr. Ling (radiation therapy) will see the patient in approximately 1 to 2 month's time.*

cc: *Dr. J. Jones, Hematology/Oncology*
Dr. W. Smith, Primary Care
Dr. M. Ling, Radiation Therapy

Result: Dr. Smith did continue to see patient for this disorder and her other chronic medical disorders with follow up as planned.

Bottom Line: The patient is the ultimate winner in a thorough report from one doctor-colleague to another.

In the following instance, two consultants left a PCP out of the loop on a patient's care.

Example of Uncoordinated Care

A healthy 45-year-old woman had routine pelvic as part of general exam with question of fibroid. Stool guaiac was negative. A gynecological consultant was asked to confirm the diagnosis. In addition to confirming the diagnosis, a positive stool guaiac was found. Without discussion with the PCP, the patient was referred to a gastroenterologist. Colonoscopy and gastroscopy were carried out, both negative. The primary care physician was informed by the patient and by letter from the gastroenterologist after the fact, the letter addressed to the referring gynecologist.

Result: Nothing was done in giving feedback to colleagues.

Bottom Line: Prevention might include a joint specialty-primary care focus group to review consequences in the process of care, and negotiate the boundaries between specialty and primary care.

On Shared Decision-Making

In the dispensary men learn to work together in groups.... Working in groups means something more than sitting in adjacent rooms. It means knowing when to call in another man and when not to occupy him unnecessarily. It means the ability to teach and to learn with the group so that it becomes constantly better knit — a faster as well as a more accurate team.

Richard C. Cabot,
The Training of the Physician, 1916[57]

Do not judge your confreres by the reports of patients, well meaning perhaps, but often strangely and sadly misrepresenting.

William Osler[58]

Shared Decision-Making

Of new importance in the doctor-patient relationship is the movement toward shared decision-making between doctors and patients, a movement which arose from the ethical-legal efforts of the 1960s to assure patient autonomy with informed consent. At first the focus was on life-threatening issues (DNR, CPR), but shifted to ordinary treatment decisions such as those for benign prostatic hypertrophy, hypertension, breast carcinoma, and even for getting tested (PSA, C-125, or bone scan).

Today, shared decision-making of another kind occurs among professionals — between physicians, between PCP and consultant, consultant and PCP, PCP and nurse practitioner. Although this process is the presumed historical practice among doctors, professional exchange about patients is wider than ever before, and especially notable in clinical teamwork and group practice. Here, shared decision-making (among MDs, RNs, NPs, PAs, SWs) with its negotiated process is more common in the management of patients with multiple chronic disorders.

Occasionally, this decision-making process breaks down. For example, the consultant's style may be overly authoritative, one of maintaining an exclusive professional autonomy in patient care so that he/she does not seek contact with referring physician or PCP before, during, or sometimes, even after treatment consultation. Whether in a one-to-one professional relationship or team context, physicians must regularly share the decision-making process.

Some special instances are notable. Consultant and practitioner are most likely to be in face-to-face communication in the hospital over acute diagnosis and treatment of the patient. The shared decision-making of PCPs with their consultants is probably most frequent in this setting, e.g., to operate or not, to use test procedures, etc.

In ambulatory practices where the long-term management of chronic illness takes place, practitioners and consultants may not be in immediate contact. Thus, PCPs may share decision-making with consultants less often. In particular, physicians may not address head on the question of who provides continuing long-term care of a patient's chronic illnesses — with the result that the consultant often "takes over" long-term management as a normative expectation or entitlement. When the patient's co-morbid disorders are numerous, shared decisions about who will manage what treatment features are important. Open discussions make for shared management that better meets the needs of patients and practitioners (as shown in Fig. 13). An example of what may result when consultation takes place without shared management is all too clear.

Here's an example of how a PCP updates a specialist on a patient whose care they share.

Consultation with Shared Management

> Dear Jim,
>
> I saw Mr. F.A. and found him without complaints. BP was 140/80, rate NSR, 70. His pacemaker is functioning normally. I will see him in one year. He is to see you soon.
>
> Sincerely, F.M.

Result: PCP's information letters to patient were also exchanged by PCP to specialist.

Bottom Line: "Best practices" of modern medicine include physicians who respect and inform one another — physicians who always keep the patient's needs at the center of any communication.

Here's an example of how a specialist and a PCP failed a patient.

Example of Consultation without Shared Management

A forty-eight-year-old woman with rheumatoid arthritis was referred to rheumatology because NSAIDs no longer adequately control her pain and joint problems. The primary care doctor had hoped the specialist would recommend a more successful therapy, and indeed, the patient was started on methotrexate with very good results. The PCP was informed of this new treatment course by letter. However, the patient now saw the rheumatologist every two months, gradually losing contact with her primary care physician. Communication was not maintained, and important general health issues such as her long struggle with obesity and Type 2 diabetes and routine gynecologic care were unattended.

Response: The PCP did not ask for regular follow-up notes from the consultant, nor were return visits directed and encouraged by the consultant.

Bottom Line: A conversation between the consultant and the PCP, directed to the common goal of comprehensive care, is needed here to ensure the patient's long-term health.

Conflicts in Consultation

"...it should be emphasized that under no circumstances, however goading they may be, should the doctor ever disparage a colleague's work or opinion, whether he be a consultant or general practitioner; and again the doctor should never belittle the service or work done by a professional institution — to the patient."

D. T. C. Barlow, British General Practice
A personal guide for students, 1973[59]

...and never listen to a story about the carelessness and inefficiency of Dr. Blank. Shut him or her up, knowing full well that the same tale may be told of you a few months later.

William Osler[58]

Colleague Criticism

In everyday patient encounters, physicians should address issues of care and treatment without criticism about colleague competence. But doctors too often fall short of this basic etiquette (see following example).

For instance, off-handed comments such as "My gosh, that's not the way he should have treated you" or "Your doctor should have referred you to a cardiologist" suggest mistaken care. Without careful analysis of a patient's care, consultant's glib patient-directed opinions about "your doctor" and his/her competence are inappropriate. These comments can seriously impede that care. In surveys of patient satisfaction, respondents report that such unprofessional comments upset them.

Questions do arise about treatment decisions, but it is better to acknowledge, as so often is true, that there are different options for intervention. Thus, a consultant should direct his/her communication directly to the patient's doctor. Patients make poor intermediaries for the criticisms one doctor may direct at another.

Here's how a consultant disparages a PCP to a patient.

An Example of Doctor-Doctor Criticism

Mrs. J suffered chest pains that her family doctor, after a full hour examination and routine testing including an EKG, had diagnosed as panic attack. After carefully explaining the diagnosis and offering appropriate treatment, the doctor was informed by the patient that she wanted a second opinion by a cardiologist. The cardiologist ordered ETT and PFTs, both normal, but in the process of evaluation remarked that those tests should have been ordered by the generalist, thus inspiring further anxiety and erosion in the primary care-patient relationship. Mrs. J then self-referred to another internist.

Result: The cardiologist never contacted the PCP.

Bottom Line: A physician who has concerns about a colleague's judgment could request that a third person mediate a conversation between the two colleagues.

Conflicts in Care

Another common conflict involves care for patients with a terminal illness. In such situations, professional differences are not uncommon. Physicians may debate, for example, whether extensive diagnostic testing will alter outcome and management, or whether the patient might be better cared for by alternative services, e.g., hospice, home care, or office-home care. Resolving such professional differences effectively demands that the entire clinical team hold family-patient confer-

ences and, as much as possible, adhere to patients' advanced care directives, proxies, and/or current preferences.

Comparisons of Care

Patients, not the consultants, may bring up dissatisfaction with their referring or primary care doctors. Consultants may learn that the patient "really can't talk" to his/her primary care physician, and wants recommendations for a referral to "another MD." Primary care physicians who "cover" the practice of colleagues on weekends or vacations may also hear similar comments and requests for "another MD."

There are no easy answers to such requests. One suggestion might be to encourage the patient to discuss dissatisfactions with the doctor — a communication seldom attempted, but one that often repairs the dissatisfaction. Another suggestion might be arriving at consensus among group practitioners or staff, that in a consumer culture, patients may want to change doctors. A physician could then offer the patient that option through the group practice plan. Still another particular involves so-called "difficult patients." Finding a staff member who will accept the care of the patient with special needs is sometimes difficult.

Uses of Doctor-Doctor and Doctor-Patient Letters

Consultants-to-MD Letters, Sent on to Patients Consultants customarily write letters to referring MDs that include advice, study results, treatment choices, and recommendations. Important additions might include information that the consultant communicated to the patient. At the discretion of the PCP, consultant letters can be sent on to patients to reinforce the shared advice of both physicians. In other instances, consultant writers may specify that the letter is only for the doctor, e.g., "Physician copy, for your records, not for redisclosure."

Consultant-to-Patient Letters, Sent to PCP Sometimes consultants write letters to patients with copies to referring MD, if consensus exists on diagnosis, treatment, and prognosis (Fig. 13). The

PCP might view the consultant's decision to write directly to the patient as a breach of professional exchange. However, with greater patient participation in the decision-making process, such letters can promote shared decision-making among the consultant, the PCP, and the patient. Moreover, the consultant's letter can reinforce the need for PCP care.

> Dear Ms. Sims:
>
> A report back to you that your colonoscopy was normal as were your stool tests. Hope you continue your improvement. And remember to get your general check-up with Dr. Smith.
>
> Sincerely,
> J. Brown, M.D.
>
> cc: Dr. Smith

> Mr. John Hay
> 18 Beach Street
> Dorchester, MA 02134
>
> Dear Mr. Hay:
>
> Just a quick note to inform you that the polyps removed during your recent colonoscopy were benign. Your condition does not require routine follow up with us. However, you should continue to see your primary care physician, Dr. Bush, for your regular check-ups.
>
> Sincerely,
> Paul Brown, M.D.
>
> cc: Dr. Samuel Bush

Figure 13 Consultant-to-Patient Letters, Sent on to PCP

PCPs can send letters about a patient's test results and exams to consultant colleagues engaged in co-management of some of the patient's problems — with, of course, the consent of the patient (Fig. 14).

Mrs. Mary Cutler
145 Boston Street #105
Revere, MA 02113

Dear Mrs. Cutler:

A note back on your blood studies you had done here on 10-29. Your blood sugar was 180, pretty stable as you have been in the past. Your creatinine or kidney function test was normal at 0.8 as was your BUN at 23, normal for kidney function. Your serum salts were all good with a sodium of 143 and a potassium of 3.5, with a chloride of 102.

Next, looking at your hemoglobin AIC, it shows that your blood sugar over the last two months has been in the average of 144 and that's good. Compliments to you.

Our best wishes to you from all the staff. We are sending these results to Dr. Smith, whom you will be seeing next about your arthritis.

Sincerely,
Barbara George, N.P.
Frank Jones, M.D.

cc: Dr. Mark Smith

Figure 14 Primary Care Physician-to-Patient Letter (Sent on to Consultants)

Follow-Up Letters, PCP to Consultants Due to emerging managed care trends which limit the number of consultations with specialists to " 1-visit," "2-visits," "3-visits," etc., the PCP has new obligations to inform the consultant of patient outcomes that previously the consultant would see on continuing or follow-up visits (Fig. 15).

Follow-up to Consultant

Mrs. G, with known coronary artery disease and a previous myocardial infarction, presented with swollen legs for three days. Physical exam confirmed warm edema, bilateral to mid-calf, without the signs of phlebitis or of congestive heart failure. Color-flow doppler studies were normal. Superficial phlebitis was considered the diagnosis and reviewed with a vascular surgeon. Follow-up CT of abdomen to exclude intra-abdominal cause was recommended.

CT was negative and phlebitis resolved in two weeks on aspirin. A letter was dispatched to consultant.

> Dear Bill:
> Just a note that the CT on Mrs. Gray was negative and her phlebitis resolved in two weeks.
>
> Best wishes,
> Dave Jones, M.D.

Figure 15 Follow-Up Letter from PCP to Consultant

Doctors as Patients of Doctors

All members of the profession, including apothecaries as well as physicians and surgeons, should be attended gratuitously…

T. Percival
Medical Ethics, 1802[44]

If a doctor is doctoring a doctor,
Does the doctor doing the doctoring
Doctor the doctor being doctored
The way the doctor being doctored
Wants to be doctored
Or does the doctor doctoring the doctor
Doctor the doctor being doctored
The way the doctoring doctor usually doctors?

Donald R. Lipsett
The Doctor as Patient, 1975[60]

Fiscal Relationships

Since physicians' own health care is covered by health insurance these days, "courtesy care" of doctors as patients seems antiquated. Rather than not charging a fee, physicians may want to take a more pragmatic approach and charge their colleagues (and families) standard fees, not to exceed what is covered by insurance. In 1993, nearly all doctors extended this modern professional courtesy to other doctors, 12% writing off the entire charge and 75% accepting insurance reimbursement as full payment.[61]

A group consensus on charging is a realistic approach, as is negotiating with "the patient-colleague."

Therapeutic Relationships

Countless books, journals and other periodicals explore in detail how doctors doctor their patients. Doctors' biases of class, gender, race, and age; their diagnoses (or lack thereof) of patients and communication with them; doctors' economic incentives in ordering tests or doing operations; their attitudes toward patients with chronic illnesses — these issues will never fail to fascinate. And while patients and public may view doctors as "never getting sick" or disabled, doctors know doctors do get sick — often "stretched out," depressed with the stress of everyday life and work of care, sometimes, too, engaged in drugs and alchohol, and, like others "come down" with one of many chronic diseases in society.[62, 63] Yet little is recorded about what the doctor himself/herself is like as a patient. Most information about treating colleague doctors is anecdotal, coming from practitioners.[64-66]

Many unwritten, informal accounts and a few formal ones about doctors-as-patients report on the doctor-patient's reluctance and delay in seeking medical aid. According to these accounts, many doctors practice self-treatment — searching for informal medical advice, getting their own consultants, ordering their own tests. One could interpret these behaviors to mean that doctors are reluctant but "informed health care consumers." Regardless, no one can specify the appropriate relationship for care of all doctors-as-patients. Because of the many uncertainties in doctor-doctor relationships and roles, negotiating the care of colleagues is most essential.

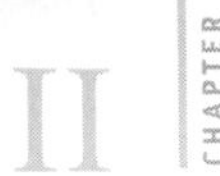

On Manager-Staff Interactions

Health care systems generally are increasing physician involvement in their governance and management in an effort to form partnerships with physicians.

Personal Communication
Hospital Administrator to Authors, 1999

...both doctors and hospital administrators often reported that doctors were not very involved in efforts to assess and change care. Doctors seem left out of the central decision-making process — apparently either by their own choice or the choice of the hospital administration. Even in hospitals espousing principles of continuous quality improvement or participatory management, doctors were rarely involved actively in efforts to improve the patient's experience.

Thomas L. Delbanco,
Through the Patient's Eyes,
Understanding and Promoting Patient-Centered Care, 1994[67]

Doctor/Physician-Manager Relationships

With managed care, more and more physicians move into administrative roles,[68] making the relationship between physician-managers and practitioners an evolving one. Managers at the present moment, and perhaps for the foreseeable future, gain authority and control — and practitioners lose out.

The expansion of managers into medicine brings a host of challenges unlike those the medical field faced earlier in the century. Business school faculties, concerned with the efficiency and organization of work, helped provide solutions by extensively studying managerial-worker relationships. Less examined tensions also simmer in the hospital and in group practices, where the obligations and goals of physician-managers and physician-practitioners may be distinct and in conflict.[69] Managers may seek to control practitioners with regulations that the latter find burdensome, or they may limit resources that practitioners regard as essential.[70,71]

The physician-manager faces conflicts in sorting through appropriate goals. He/she must decide whether to allow physician-practitioner participation in HMO and capitation contract negotiations, for instance. Serving as the bridge between practitioners who provide care and insurers who pay for it can make the physician-manager feel like a tightrope artist without a net. Of course, this situation did not exist when patients and doctors played more individualistic roles in health care.

In the new market, however, the assumption that physician-managers will always identify with the "practicing doc" because of their own medical education and continued part-time practice (already diminished from 50% to 10% or less in the last 10 years)[72] is unlikely. Managers, physicians or not, become the new elite of practice organizations, deciding on appropriate manpower, fiscal resources, and organizational information for providing health care.

Relationships between the practitioner and physician-manager produce tension when the former discerns that the latter acts without engaging fellow practitioners in decision-making. For example, administrators recently dropped senior staff from a hospital's practice organization without discussion.

Yet the physician-manager can also engage doctors, whether individually or as a group, for the goal of improved care and treatment — not just to improve the "bottom line." Health care management literature extols, after all, the importance of practitioner participation in the design of quality measures, "pathways" of treatment and clinical outcomes.[73,74]

One can frame managerial communications about goals in two different lights. A manager could ask a group of physicians a broad question about an issue that affects them all: "What do you think about the hospital stays for condition X? Can we review these?" Or, to the individual practitioner, the manager might be more direct — even critical — about a particular issue. "Your patients' stays are too long. What are you going to do about them?" Some practitioners experience anger and shame upon receiving criticism from a colleague with more authority, reacting with resistance instead of cooperation. That the manager possesses strong communication skills matters greatly.

No one can chart the future of physician-manager/practitioner relationships as the market economy of health care expands. Concerns of efficiency, growth, and profits will likely drive those who enter administrative jobs — despite the history of hospitals and medical practices as nonprofit enterprises. The professionalism of the doctor will be tested and stretched. Expectations of cost control in care and treatment will serve as the "turning point" around which the patient, the plan (or the public), the organization, the insurer, and the practitioner revolve.[75]

On Hospitalists, Case Managers, and Others

Two new positions have emerged in the hospital under managed care and will increasingly become part of outpatient practices: (1) the hospitalist and (2) the case manager. While one trained as a doctor and the other as a nurse (or nurse practitioner), both play important roles in managing care and containing costs. Each adds as well to the division and control of medical work, the differential status of professionals, and the complexity of interprofessional communication.[76]

Hospitalists are often recently graduated medical residents and fellows or more senior internists with subspecialty training.[77-79] They serve as the "in-house" attending physician (the "physician of record") for the patients of community-based PCPs (who are absent from daily hospital care). Or they care for particular patients of PCPs, such as cardiac patients whose hospital management has been assigned to cardiology. In brief, hospitalists oversee, evaluate, and manage the daily care of in-patients; they decide on length-of-stay and discharge plans, whether to home or to care at other institutions.[80]

Hospitalists could share their decisions with community-based PCPs by maintaining daily contact by phone, facsimile, and electronic mail. So far, however, studies do not document whether or how hospitalists communicate with PCPs other than through a patient's discharge summary.

Case managers, as nurses or nurse practitioners, coordinate home care services and alternative care facilities that patients may require on discharge. Knowledgeable about options in the "continuum of care" (acute care, sub-acute nursing facilities, short-stay nursing homes, rehabilitation hospitals, home care, day care), case managers organize the transfer of hospitalized patients into less costly settings. And, working in out-patient practices, they also organize community-based home services (IV therapies, physical therapy, medical devices, visits by home-health aides).

Both hospitalists and case managers, by the nature of their jobs, need to communicate closely with PCPs, specialists, residents and support staff. In straightforward cases of patient care, communication may need only involve a summary of decisions made and transmitted to various professionals, institutions, and agencies. More complicated cases, however, may compel a hospitalist or case manager to exchange views with PCPs about patients and together resolve questions and/or conflicts about treatment.

Both of these managerial positions break tradition with longstanding professional roles.

Hospitalists may end the era of continuity of care in which a patient's PCP or personal physician provides care in both hospital and office settings. At the same time, hospitalists may also create new organizational status in the profession, diminishing the role of the practicing PCP. A new "continuum of care"— defined by multiple settings and changing staffs, and administered by hospitalists and case managers — may increasingly substitute for the PCP.

Among other roles, the case manager also replaces in part the medical social worker. A focus on the patient's psychosocial adjustment to illness may no longer prevail as the case manager arranges for less expensive care. Overall, decision-making at the site of care in order to speed up treatment and save money further divides medical work — a process that began with disease specialization. No one can predict whether the new managers and PCPs will continue to seek each other

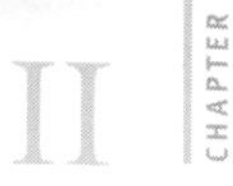

out or whether the input of the latter will remain of primary importance in patient care.

Mistakes, Impairments and Roles

"The doctor is constantly tested by results. He is repeatedly brought to book...Many of his mistakes cannot be covered up. This, like the burdens of responsibility and the calls to all around resourcefulness, is a great developer of any good that may be in him."

Richard C. Cabot
The Effect of Doctoring on the Doctor, 1922[81]

"The goal should be extreme safety. But we cannot reach that goal through exhortation, censure, outrage, and shame. We can reach it only by commitment to change, so that normal human errors can be made irrelevant to outcome, continually found, and skillfully mitigated. So long as it involves humans — and thank God it does — health care will never be free of errors. But it can be free of injury."

Donald M. Berwick
Not Again!
Preventing Errors Lies in Redesign — Not Exhortation, 2001[82]

Professional Mistakes

Data confirm old ideas that professional "mistakes" are common.[83,84] Some "mistakes" go to court; litigation means that the physician(s) and nurses involved are not supposed to discuss the issue among colleagues. Unfortunately, many "mistakes" remain with the doctor and nurse who so often have no place to go to share their shame or grief in not meeting high standards of care.[85] Talking about mistakes is difficult even

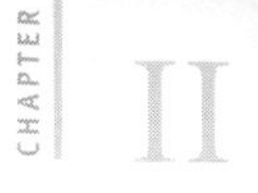

with oneself. Shared discussions with trusted colleagues can be of great benefit, and colleagues should be accessible for such support.[86-88]

Impairments and Sickness

In addition to commenting on interprofessional relationships in the context of patient care, teaching, and education, the authors of this manual hope to generate discussion about another, rather sensitive context — namely, the impact of personal problems on the doctor-doctor relationship.

The impairments of colleagues by psychiatric illness, medical disorders, substance abuse, or physical disabilities may influence one's relationships with and acceptance of them.[81] Indeed, the onset of illness and disablement may lead to indifference and rejection. As colleagues we should accept and support fellow practitioners with impaired behaviors and illnesses, encouraging them to seek appropriate help from their personal physicians and/or physician assistance committees (available both in our staff organizations and outside in our medical societies).[89,90] Acceptance and support make for meaningful solidarity.

Meeting Behaviors

Hospital and teaching services hold numerous (some would say redundant) meetings to review patient care: "morning report," "chief rounds," morbidity-mortality ("M and M") conferences, tumor boards, team meetings for managing practice capitation. In these meetings, "chief rounds," for example, the chair may not set appropriate limits. Residents may "scapegoat the privates" who handle patients less sensitively than the physicians-in-training who are new, and strangers at the patient's bedside.[91,92] Divisive comments can emerge. "Generalist docs are good, except when the patient becomes sick," or, "Doctor X keeps every patient that gets referred."

Elsewhere, senior residents under pressure for efficiency may derisively "dump on" junior residents and medical students who are slow in getting the work-up and "scut work" done. Shamed rather than mentored, students in response remain quiet but less enthusiastic colleagues.

Departmental chairpersons, attending physicians, residents, and group practice staff must help set a problem-solving and learning tone to meetings. Everyone present must focus on cooperative, constructive behavior in discussion of patients' care.

Doctor-Resident Relationships

To promote the welfare of the patients in the ward or out-patient clinic to which they are assigned is the Residents' and House Officers' first concern. In the care of such patients they are responsible for carrying out the directions of the staff.

Charles Short
Regulations for Residents and House Officers
MGH, 1931[93]

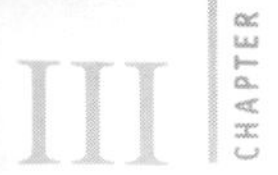

Residents and Supervision

Once upon a time, residents worked as apprentices under the direction of the staff — and under the assumption that they must always do what they were told. Clinical directions did not change after their daily contact with attending staff. Today, technical interventions alter the above scenario. Medical conditions move very fast compared to the old watchful waiting for the resolution of acute illness.

Take the once prescribed six-week bed rest for acute myocardial infarct compared with today's interventions that change hourly with clot lysis treatment followed by angiogram, angioplasty, and/or stents. As a result of rapid changes in patients' disorders and needs for prompt treatment interventions, the staff-to-apprentice relationship is no longer a directive one but one of shared decision-making. Residents, although still in training, perform as junior staff. Moreover, schooled in our modem culture of equality and self-advocacy, they expect an egalitarian teacher-student exchange (as in Harvard Medical School's New Pathway program).[94] This method of learning and problem-solving affects how residents perform the tasks of care: they are able and expected to define diagnostic problems quickly and organize the sequence of diagnostic testing and treatment.

Furthermore, physicians-in-training today are, compared to earlier times, often at a more advanced stage of personal-professional development. Many share lives with spouses or significant others and devote themselves not only to medicine but also to raising a family (another increasingly egalitarian role). And with medical technology developing at a rapid pace, younger physicians may more comfortably use diagnostic and treatment technologies in patient care than some of their seniors.

In the modern hospital and clinic where they train, residents expect to take "therapeutic responsibility" for clinical work and, in turn, to receive the appropriate rewards. Senior staff, of course, must supervise, teach, coach, precept and mentor residents — acknowledging all the while that residents co-care for patients with them and deserve compliments and face-to-face thanks for their work. Changes in residents' medical education and clinical organization, as well as in technologies used, thus make the old apprenticeship model of medical training antiquated. Training supervision, less directive and more participatory than in years past, may lead to exchanges once unheard of between senior staff and residents. For example, negotiating responsibility for a patient may occur and the exchange of evidence-based medicine.

Patients on the "teaching wards" are no longer strangers unattached to PCPs in the community or on the hospital staff. Increasingly, these patients come under the care of PCPs in the hospital's network; therefore, PCPs and residents must share decision-making autonomy and therapeutic responsibility for them. Similarly, a patient in the "private service" requires more constant attention of resident physicians, who in turn share decisions with the patient's private physician.

Frequent interactions with a physician-in-training may result in a patient identifying with that resident rather than the attending physician. Writing in the 1980s, Cassell noted that therapeutic responsibility is enormously educational for physicians-in-training, but that it can also be difficult for the attending physician to maintain formal responsibility without participating in the patient's direct care.[95] The physician-in-training may also find it hard to remain receptive to accepting the directions and experience the attending has to offer.[96]

Unfortunately, differences in practice styles (often dependent on how recently the attending physician received his/her training) may blind a resident to the broad perspective and wisdom of a senior physician while evidence-based medicine brings them together.

Regardless of the changes in the nature of medical education, training, and the trainees themselves, residents will always need mentoring by senior physicians. Managed care programs won't change that.[97] No technology, after all, no matter how advanced, can substitute for the transmittal of sound judgment from one generation of physicians to the next. Senior and junior physicians must learn anew to work together; changes in federal law deem that they must.

The Health Care Financing Administration (HCFA) recently redefined the relationship between the teaching physician (the "attending") and resident by changing regulations for Medicare payment for services provided by residents.[98] The law requires the physical presence of attending physicians during the key portion of any billable service or procedure; attendings must also document their involvement with a short record note. These changes follow the HCFA's well publicized audit and fine of the University of Pennsylvania, which had billed for services under the names of attending physicians when residents actually performed the services.

Still other changes in ambulatory supervision include: (1) attendings can precept no more than four residents a session, (2) cannot see their own patients during the session, and (3) must attest that they reviewed and agreed upon the evaluation-management plan with the resident; in addition, (4) attendings must assume management responsibility for patients seen by residents.

These changes mark an important departure in the resident's autonomy and relationship to senior attending physicians. Historically, prior to Medicare's contribution to teaching, hospital staff regarded resident physicians as: (1) staff who provided office care to outpatients without supervision, (2) staff who provided care to non-private ward patients under supervision of an attending physician, and (3) staff who assisted the private staff in the care of their private hospitalized patients.

Beginning in the late 1960s, when Medicare Part B payment for residency training began, teaching hospitals involved the attending physician in the care of individual Medicare patients. This led to an almost parallel system of care by residents who ran the "Residents' Ward Service" and their outpatient clinics with varying amounts of senior physician oversight. Today, with less independence and greater supervision, residents must learn to care for patients in a team model in which attending physicians immerse themselves in all aspects of the patient's care. No longer should residents search for autonomy in therapeutic responsibility, as physicians everywhere must share and negotiate care.

Similarly, in the case of surgery, the pyramidal five-year residency derived from Hopkins, Pennsylvania, and the Massachusetts General Hospital[99] may need retooling. Confining decision-making to the residency staff itself with regard to "ward patients," thus avoiding external supervision, control, surveillance, or participation of the private practice senior staff (except the Chief of Service), no longer seems feasible. Meanwhile, managed care programs, public or private, continue to review the care of all their patients externally — even if this process is not done internally.

Specifics in Resident Staff Care

The Attending Physician must be kept informed of any serious development in his patient's condition and must approve of all forms of treatment. The House Officer acts as assistant to the Attending Physician; the responsibility for the patient's care rests with the latter.

Regulations for Residents and House Staff
MGH, 1938[93]

As attending physician, you are responsible and accountable for all patient care decisions and actions by the housestaff on your team. This includes responsibility for all errors of omission and commission by housestaff, as well as their documentation and medical record keeping responsibilities.

You should be readily accessible to participate in diagnostic and management decisions for the patients on your service at all times.

Guidelines for Attending Physicians
University of Washington Medical Center, 2001

Sanando docemus (healing we teach) — today, one another, residents and staff.

For residents, hospital care today means caring for patients as a joint enterprise with senior staff, even when the staff places residents under the supervision of an attending or staff physician. From a patient's admission to discharge, the resident evaluates the patient, orders tests, interprets data, makes treatment decisions, arranges consults, and often decides which level of care — ward, intensive care unit, or subspecialty floor — best suits a patient's needs.

Residents sometimes perform these decisions and tasks under close staff supervision, especially in settings such as the emergency ward or intensive care unit where full-time attendings are available for co-managing and consulting. On the wards, however, and during evening hours and weekends, residents will function with independence and less direct supervision.

Just as identification (on the cover of the chart) of the patient's attending physician (PCP or subspecialist) is essential for optimizing care, so is identification, in a similar fashion, of the house staff who is responsible for that patient. This is particularly important for facilitating communication between residents and attending physicians when services are large and residents numerous. Communication, after all, is no longer about "my patient" but "our patient."

The resident's on-call shift is invariably filled with myriad unsupervised decisions about the patient's care. Which decisions and results need to be negotiated with, and communicated to, the attending physician can be determined by the resident by asking himself/herself several questions: (1) What are appropriately and necessarily supervised, shared decisions? (2) What are simple courtesies to the patient's attending physician? (3) What are the medicolegal ramifications of bad outcomes?

From the resident's perspective, no guidelines clearly address what circumstances require a call to the attending. And attending physicians vary in their need and desire for involvement or for information. No one argues about the extremes. If a patient becomes critically unstable, the need for close resident-staff communication is clear. A less dramatic but still serious patient condition may also provoke anxiety for staff physician and resident alike around decision-making initiatives. Finally, decisions initiated in a perfunctory fashion that result in poor outcomes foster ill will between residents and staff. Shared decision-making between senior staff and junior staff over not only the goals but also the content of care is a necessity today. Some items for shared communication and negotiated decisions include:

Staff to Resident

- **Rationale for hospitalization** and details of prior care
- **Information about the patient** as a person and the patient's family (as staff so often has long-term contact with patient)
- **Goals of care or referral**
- **Diagnostic testing**, its appropriateness given the particulars of the case
- **Consultations**
- **Coverage of patient's care** in staff's absence
- **Communication** of end-of-life decisions, their parameters

Resident to Staff

- **Acute changes** in patient's medical condition (see example on next page)
- **Information** about diagnostic tests for immediate decisions
- **Patient's death**, immediate reporting

Here, a resident calls late about a deteriorating patient.

Example of Failure to Report Acute Changes in Patient's Medical Condition

Mr. X had been admitted two days earlier for CHF. The resident saw him at 2:00 a.m. for increasing SOB, began treating him for CHF, but also began the process of further evaluation which included transfusing the patient for a low hematocrit, and getting blood gases, a CXR, EKG, and enzymes. The patient's condition was slightly improved after diuresis and 02. By 6:00 a.m., however, the patient again had difficulty. At this point, the resident considered a pulmonary embolism and began to negotiate the necessary radiological procedures which, in fact, demonstrated a large left-sided pulmonary embolus. The attending physician was called at 6:30 a.m. When she arrived on the wards at 9:00 a.m. she let the resident know that he should have called earlier when the diagnosis was in question.

Comment: Such feedback is not regularly practiced.

Resident-to-Resident Relationships

While in residency training, physicians first learn the status of physician-physician relationships. In learning to care for patients, new residents interact with one another, with more senior residents and fellows, and with their attending physicians. Although no longer based on a competitive pyramidal promotion system, training programs still contain inevitable competitive and hierarchical features. Second- and third-year residents assume responsibility for the work of the first-year residents on their teams and under their tutelage. In turn, of course, all residents answer to the attending physician-of-record.

Resident physicians, as their training proceeds, seek greater therapeutic responsibility, a search for autonomy that may prevent them from asking for help and guidance from supervising staff. While initial interactions between residents and staff physicians resemble the relationship between students and teachers, over three years of training a new, more equal relationship evolves. The resident increasingly becomes a collaborative physician, a peer who works well in groups both in the hospital and outside of it.

Modern care of the patient requires closer teamwork among physicians-in-training than ever before. Shorter, structured work hours, night float systems, off-ward assignments such as ambulatory practice sessions and specialty rotations make the resident's training more tolerable and diverse, but still stressful.[100-102] At the same time, these progressive changes in physician training take the individual house officer away from the hour-to-hour, bedside management of the acutely ill patient.

By necessity, team members who care simultaneously for a patient must share such tasks as evaluation and therapeutic responsibility. Knowledge transmission, task coordination, and cross-cover obligations comprise a new list of social skills required of and learned by the resident.

Shared responsibilities within a team of physicians-in-training define resident-resident interactions. Coordinated patient care requires good communication skills, the ability to work interdependently with others, talent in organizing care, and a willingness to ask for or accept help. With multiple rotations on hospital services, teams come and go, in which personal relationships may not be repeated in the three years of training.

First-year residents sign out their patients to each other. No longer does one resident have total responsibility for the care of a patient. Going "off duty" means shared decision-making with cross-covering colleagues. The degree of closeness among residents, how much they may like, trust or respect one another, certainly varies. Physicians-in-training may experience conflict over workloads unevenly distributed, decisions improperly made — a covering resident initiates treatment, for instance, about which the patient's primary resident later disagrees — or when communication breaks down.

Given the stressful demands of responsibility and collaboration in patient care, Messner advises that residents' "resilience can be enhanced" by discussions of their experience with supervisors or in Balint groups.[103, 104]

Specific Lessons of Hospital Care

On-Call Coverage

The usual evening scenario for the team (a senior/junior resident and two or more interns) is to "sign out" to a team member, the on-call resident. The on-call resident is responsible for the night-time care of patients and admissions. During the "sign out," departing residents review with the on-call resident information about patients, events of the day, studies pending, evolving symptoms and signs, and preparations for the next day — often aided by a detailed work sheet. The next morning, the on-call resident presents new admissions and updates the team on patients covered throughout the night.

Night Float Coverage

Most residency programs now use "night floats," in which a resident covers a service for new patient admissions from early evening until the following morning. The "night float" resident then transfers the patient to the usual medical team for ongoing care. Most properly, this transfer occurs on morning work rounds; the night float resident presents the patient to the entire medical team, introduces the patient to any "new doctors" responsible for care, and transfers direct care to another resident.

Emergency Ward Transfer

Upon evaluating, treating and admitting patients to the hospital, emergency ward residents should formally transfer care of the patient to medical team residents in person. The emergency ward resident should introduce the patient to the medical team resident; together the residents should review the evaluation and management of the patient in the emergency ward. Courtesy and shared learning also mean that the medical team resident should provide follow-up to his/her emergency ward colleague on the outcome of the patient.

Service-to-Service Transfers

Patients often stabilize in one acute setting (a medical cardiac intensive care unit, for instance) and then require transfer to a less acute setting (such as a step-down unit or medical ward). Residents responsible for these transfers should provide a summary or transfer note that details previous events of care. They should also communicate this information in person to the accepting resident. Moreover, residents who accept the transferred patient onto the new service should meet the patient prior to transfer. Similarly, transfers from one service, such as medicine, to another specialty, such as surgery or neurology, also require detailed transfer notes and person-to-person communication to facilitate shared care.

Resident Learning in Ambulatory Care

Compared to learning-to-care for hospital patients, the conditions for residents' learning-to-care for outpatients has different organization, workload incentive, and patient characteristics.

The first difference is in clinical organization. In the hospital, the resident works in a practice-teaching organization where he/she is one of a team of doctors with a collective responsibility for a group of patients, supervised by an attending. In the clinic, the resident, by contrast, is a member of a small practice team of nurse practitioners, registered nurses, other residents, and senior staff (some as supervisors), but he/she attends his/her ambulatory patients as an individual practitioner with supervisory backup.

Second, the number of patients admitted by others in the hospital, ranging from EW and senior hospital physicians to clinic and health center staffs, determines the workload-incentive of the resident. In the hospital, residents attend the intake of new admissions and participate in whatever continuing care patients require. Not only do residents exert little control over this system, but they must also face incentives to fill beds and demands to see new acute cases. In contrast, responsibility for the workload incentive in the clinic, in large part, belongs to the resident him/herself. The resident schedules patients into his/her own practice session, accommodating return visits as well as new patients seeking appointments.

The resident's incentives for a full outpatient workload vary with his/her own incentives for a busy schedule. Departmental priorities for scheduling patients for care play a role, but so may a resident's concerns that care and learning in the clinic not conflict with hospital duties, limiting his/her intake of new patients.

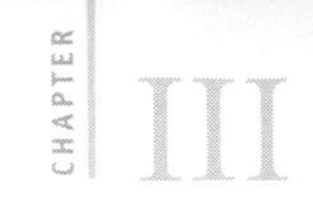

Third, patients' illnesses vary in hospital and outpatient settings, eliciting, in turn, different learning incentives. Unlike the acute new illnesses of the hospitalized patient, the outpatient clinic often brings scheduled patients with known chronic illnesses, attendant psychosocial distress and multiple co-morbid disorders. Health promotion, disease-disability management, and prevention goals that require an emphasis on screening early diagnosis and behavioral change are major tasks of outpatient learning for the resident. Given these differences in organization, workload, and patients' disorders, outpatient learning requires more commitment by the resident to creating his/her own learning-practice experiences.

Supervision in Ambulatory Care

Different models of staff supervision characterize the ambulatory training of residents throughout modern medicine's history. In old models, residents often worked alone in "resident" or "service" clinics, caring for patients with little direct involvement of attending physicians. The attending acted more as a senior consultant than as a supervisor, promoting residents' "learning-by-doing" and clinical independence. Both provided "service" to "clinic-hospital patients" as members of the staff.

Fiscal and medical-legal demands, however, as well as the detailed managerial approach that managed care arrangements require, alter these models and resident-staff responsibilities to patients. More and more, residents and attendings must join together in the co-care of the patient; more and more, attendings are paid for supervision. From a patient-care perspective, this new arrangement may not be ideal. Such close supervision of the resident by the attending, or two-person care, is not always appropriate for nor acceptable to patients. Nonetheless, managed care may require it as a prerequisite to allowing residents to care for "their patients."

Other models require residents to present each patient, old and new, to an attending physician. The latter reviews the patient's history, re-examines the patient, checks the laboratory findings, and helps to determine management. Intermediate arrangements are also common, such as allowing the resident to decide whether to review any patient with the attending physician.

CHAPTER IV

Doctor-Student Teaching Relationships

To hold my teacher in this art equal to my own parents; to make him partner in my livelihood; when he is in need of money to share mine with him; to consider his family as my own brothers; and to teach them this art, if they want to learn it, without fee or indenture; to impart precept, oral instruction, and all other instruction to my own sons, the sons of my teacher, and to indentured pupils who have taken the physician's oath, but to nobody else.

Hippocrates

The spirit of the hospital has always been, first, to do everything it can for its patients; second, to use patients, so far as it is right and consistent with their best care, for educational purposes; third, to have its data so accurately recorded that it furnishes the maximum aid to the advancement of medical and surgical science.

Trustees, Massachusetts General Hospital
Annual Report, 1904

Teachers' Responsibilities

Teachers' responsibilities to students include imparting medical knowledge and technique, medicine's science, and imparting insight and understanding into the personal care of patients, medicine's humanism. Both are essential. For these goals, according to Stanley Reiser, physician-ethicist,[105] teachers must cultivate certain duties and behaviors:

- **Candor** Without honest feedback, students cannot know where they need to improve. Without an honest revealing of their own limits, teachers present a false image of the limits of knowledge.
- **Trust** Bestowing trust on learners encourages them to become reliable.
- **Respect** Showing respect for the diversity, effort, accomplishments, viewpoints, and limits of students gives them a dignity essential for growth and self-esteem.

Students' Responsibilities

According to Dr. Reiser, students possess the following duties toward their teachers:

- **Reciprocity** Students must recognize the need to reward their teachers' efforts with a commitment to learn.
- **Honesty** Students must not shirk from acquiring knowledge and recognizing the areas in which they need more learning.
- **Openness** Students should be receptive to new ideas and give their teachers a fair hearing.

With professional life and education increasingly centered in large organizations, staff members of all ranks should ideally reflect the above-stated values and behaviors.

Teachers, as residents, fellows, or attending physicians, instruct and observe students. In turn, students observe the performance of the teaching staff. Unfortunately, surveys 3–11 and seminar reports[106] make clear that our teaching hospital staffs, in the perception of students and residents, do not always live up to these ideals. Too often teachers fail to respect students and display less than ethical behavior.

Both students and residents report humiliating ethnic and racial discrimination from staff — senior residents, nurses, and attending physicians — and, not infrequently, sexual harassment because of gender or sexual orientation. While hospitals try to change these "behaviors" by "diversity training courses" or by creating ombudspersons, medical school teachers and hospital residency directors should be open to "feedback" from students and residents. Such openness enables the teaching staff to learn to improve not only their pedagogical performance but also their teacher-student relationships. And while feedback most often occurs through evaluation forms, check lists and commentaries delivered to program directors, face-to-face encounters between students and teachers may more effectively produce change.

Besides the formal care and learning exercises of clinical teaching in ambulatory practices, physicians can provide students and residents with relationships of another kind — as mentors or advisers, offering guidance on career decisions and development.

Department Heads' Interaction with Staff

However, the failure to distinguish between manners and morals also suggests, erroneously, that from personal virtue, acceptable social behavior will follow effortlessly. All you need is a good heart, the rest will take care of itself. You don't ever have to write thank you letters.

A standard set of manners also disguises the fact, inevitable and desirable in a democracy, that not everyone agrees on every issue.

Judith Martin
Common Courtesy[107]

Recognition of the staffs' teaching efforts by department heads and course directors is, of course, acknowledged by academic appointments. Sometimes, too, staff members receive such institutional "perks" as library privileges and free tuition to post-graduate courses. Yet the staff's voluntary supervision of patient care by students and residents often goes unpublished and remains out of sight. Paid or unpaid, these efforts of the staff should be acknowledged by personal thanks from departmental heads and course directors (Fig. 16).

THE GENERAL HOSPITAL

Dr. Mark Jones
Medical Services
The General Hospital

Dear Mark:

Thank you so much for teaching this last year in the new Core Medicine Clerkship. We are deeply appreciative of the enormous expenditure of time and effort you have made, as well as the contribution of the patients in your practice. We know this has been accomplished at the expense of other activities. You also have the enthusiastic thanks of the students for your invaluable instruction. Your commitment to care and teaching helps the Service maintain its mission and professional esprit.

Sincerely,
James Brown, M.D.
Chief, Medical Services

Figure 16 Thank You Letter to Recognize Teaching Efforts

Formal notes of other kinds that range from complimenting staff on outside community work or awards to acknowledging a retirement or career move are important too. Yet administrators and teaching physicians alike should also heed the need for kudos that are personal, those everyday ordinary acknowledgments among co-workers that sometimes get lost in our increasingly large practice organizations.

CHAPTER V

Doctor-Nurse Relationships

...Meanwhile, there will be an increasing overlap of activities between medicine and nursing, and more specialization will be demanded as new responsibilities are shifted from the doctor to the nurse.

John H. Knowles
Hospitals, Doctors and the Public Interest, 1965[108]

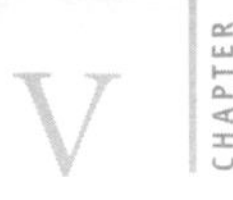

Introduction

While this manual has focused on professional relationships between doctors, these relationships, of course, have never taken place in isolation from other health care professionals. Doctors have always been part of an expanding nexus of interprofessional relationships — mostly with nurses, but also with social workers, physician assistants, physical therapists, occupational therapists, and technicians. Today, with the expansion of care outside the hospital and of team care inside, nurses and nurse practitioners undertake tasks in collaboration with, and often independently of, the doctor. Thus, nurse-doctor professional relationships, on and off the hospital campus, fall within the purview of this manual.

Practicing Together:
Participatory Management, Doctors and Nurses

Better "doctoring together" is important, yet by itself, it does not assure optimal patient care unless doctors engage other professionals in similar conduct. Just as the organization of care has changed the intraprofessional doctor-doctor relationship, so has it changed the interprofessional, e.g., nurse-doctor, relationship, as well as those with the other health professions, including the newer administrator or manager-doctor relationship, in which the administrator may make discretionary decisions without professional input or limit the discretionary decisions of the physician. In these expanding and complex interprofessional relationships, collaboration is important for optimal patient care in and outside the hospital.[109]

In the Hospital

The need for rapid intervention, the decreased length of hospital stay, the greater complexity of acute care, and the work demands on all clinicians mean that the management of the inpatient illness requires good communication between doctors and staff nurses, a shift away from the old "doctor-nurse game."[110-113] For coordinated nurse-doctor inpatient care, essential topics of communication include:

- **The patient's condition and response** to treatment
- **Treatment goals/plans** and projected time frame
- **Changes in the treatment plan**
- **Anticipated discharge needs/services**
- **Communication** with patient and family

These issues of care require communication among staff from multiple fields, with agencies outside the hospital, and with patient and family members. Interprofessional dialogue about these issues should be negotiated so both nurses and doctors can work together toward common treatment goals with patients and families. Nowadays, it is not uncommon for the nurse to be the link between the physician and other consulting staff, making nurse-doctor communication most important. Studies suggest that collaboration and coordination between physicians and nurses is responsible for better patient outcomes, including lower intensive care unit mortality rates and fewer drug errors and adverse drug reactions (including fatal ones).[114-116]

Face-to-face interactions give both doctor and nurse the opportunity to discuss the topics noted above, and also to ask questions that one may not suitably pose in the medical record. Interdisciplinary rounds also provide a forum for such discussions, but often serve primarily as teaching rounds for the house staff and medical students. At the end of the case discussion, the physician sometimes poses a brief question to a nurse, such as, "What do you need?" A more productive question might be: "Are there other concerns that haven't been raised?" or "What does the patient need?".

The hospital medical record, however, is increasingly the vehicle for communication between nurse and doctor about the patient's condition. Thus, the record needs to include more information than in the past. Thorough communication not only improves patient care, but also its efficiency, reducing the likelihood of multiple phone calls and duplication of effort that so often occur in the acute care setting. Once again, keeping the focus of the record on the patient (condition, needs, plans, goals, etc.) will facilitate patient care and ease workplace stress. Physician and nursing notes are never the place to address professional differences, or to comment on the judgment, actions or omissions of nurse or physician colleagues.

The following hospital scenario illustrates the consequences of lapses in nurse-doctor communication.

Without Follow-Through, Attending Doctor Creates Confusion

Mr. X has been told by his attending physician that he will be discharged tomorrow, that the physician will come by in the morning to give Mr. X his prescriptions and discharge instructions. The physician writes in the progress notes, "Probable discharge tomorrow," but does not complete the discharge sheet or medications. The next day the patient's wife comes at 9 a.m. in order to be there when the physician arrives. By 11 a.m., the physician has not been able to see Mr. X. The nurse cannot prepare a medication teaching booklet, nor answer his questions about medications because there is no record information on the post-hospital plan.

Meanwhile Mr. X's bed has been assigned to an Emergency Department patient. Mr. X and his wife (who is now worrying about the mounting parking fee) repeatedly ask the nurse about discharge time; they are increasingly anxious, and thereby require more real attention from the nurse. The dietary staff want to know if the patient will need lunch; the housekeeping staff want to know when the room can be cleaned; and Emergency wants to know when the bed will be ready. Given the mounting concerns, the nurse calls the physician, who estimates his arrival at around noon. By the time the physician arrives, half the nursing staff has gone to lunch. Mr. X's nurse, who has stayed on in anticipation of his discharge, is responsible for twice as many patients now, but has to prepare a teaching booklet for Mr. X, make sure that he understands his medication and follow-up instructions, as well as have him sign two forms and remove his saline lock. Mr. X is by now inattentive and impatient, the ED calls for the third time, incurring the ire of the secretary, the kitchen delivers a lunch that Mr. X will not be eating, and the housekeeping staff have had to rearrange their work in order to get the bed ready.

In the scenario above, many hospital staff members took extra time and effort, at some cost to the organization and patients (Mr. X, the waiting patient in the ED, the other patients who received less nursing attention because of extra time spent dealing with Mr. X). Had the physician written the discharge information the day before discharge, given a time estimate to Mr. X, or had his office call the unit when the doctor was delayed, much of the anxiety and extra work could have been avoided. The Admitting Office could have reassigned the ED patient and Mr. X's nurse would have reviewed the discharge instructions while Mr. X waited for the doctor and was in a less anxious frame of mind.

Here's how a nurse helped a resident avoid a major treatment mistake.

Resident-Nurse on Treatment: Prevention of Patient Decompensation

The resident wants to discontinue oxygen therapy for Mrs. Y, a frail 90-year-old with CAD and resolving pneumonia, who lives semi-independently in congregate housing. He looks at the vital sign sheet and notes that her oxygen saturation values have been in the 90s for several days. He removes her oxygen and writes an order to that effect. He then seeks out Mrs. Y's nurse to tell her of the change in therapy. Mrs. Y's nurse is surprised and comments that Mrs. Y consistently desaturates to the mid-80s when ambulating without oxygen, information that is documented on the vital sign sheet. After a short discussion, the resident decides to continue oxygen therapy with activity and to re-examine the treatment plan for Mrs. Y.

The resident had misread the vital sign sheet. Only because he talked with the nurse was he able to avoid compromising Mrs. Y's status by prematurely discontinuing oxygen. The plan to discontinue oxygen therapy might have been discussed at morning collaborative work rounds, thereby setting the stage for further resident/nurse communication about this issue. Had the intern not informed the nurse of the therapy change, she would have had to page him later to question the order, and then a cross-covering resident unfamiliar with the patient might have had to address the issue. And while various health-care professionals sorted out a decision, Mrs. Y would remain at risk.

On Treatment

A Nurse Avoids Further Patient Compromise

Mr. Z has HIV and renal failure. He receives peritoneal dialysis (PD) Q6h. He continues to fail, is anorectic and cachectic, and today is hypotensive. His attending physician, concerned that Mr. Z is hypovolemic, writes an order to "decrease PD to 1.5 %" (from 2.5 %). As the physician is leaving to write the order, he passes Mr. Z's nurse who is entering Mr. Z's room to start the 10 a.m. PD exchange, but he says nothing to her. After the exchange, the nurse fortuitously looks at Mr. Z's chart because Mr. Z had made some vague comment about "the doctor changing my dialysis." (She does not usually have time to check charts at this busy time of day, and the unit transcribers can at best check books once an hour.) The nurse notes the new PD order, drains the exchange of 2.5 % dialysate (which would have dwelled for five hours, further contributing to Mr. Z's hypovolemia), and pre-

pares a new exchange at 1.5 %. She still has to consult an MD to: 1. confirm that the medication additives to the new PD will remain the same (not specified in the order), and 2. ask the MD about the volume of the exchange, which the patient had requested be decreased because of severe abdominal discomfort, but which the attending physician did not address in his note or order.

A brief review between the doctor and nurse would have:

- **Prevented an unnecessary (and painful) PD exchange**
- **Kept the patient on his PD schedule** instead of delaying it an hour
- **Allowed for clarification** of the PD order, thereby cuing the doctor to write the complete order, including additives and volume
- **Saved the time of both the nurse and physician**, who had to talk subsequently on the phone
- **Avoided the patient's risk for exacerbated hypotension** secondary to hypovolemia

In Ambulatory Care

In group practices outside the hospital — clinics, HMOs, neighborhood health centers, faculty practices, professional corporations (IPAs) — doctors and nurse practitioners collaborate in the care of walking patients. Eighty percent of the patients live with chronic illness, making regular scheduled "return visits;" the remainder are elderly patients (many of whom come infrequently because they receive care at home from family members, home-health aides and nurses) who visit with new complaints, or are new patients to the practice.

In the office, the participatory management of long-term patients requires ongoing communication and consensus by physicians and nurses concerning:

- **Shared care by doctor and nurse**, its joint acknowledgement and reminders with patients
- **Goals of care**
- **Occurrence and diagnosis of new problems**
- **Scope of the work-up**
- **Data collected**
- **Treatment decisions**
- **Communication** with patients and families
- **Schedule of visits** or follow-up

Unlike nurse-doctor communications in the hospital, where joint usage of the medical record means that nurse and doctor do not have to meet, nurse-doctor communications in the office setting usually occur face-to-face — often with the patient present to assure joint consensus and management.

Community-Based Home Care

Doctor-nurse communication involving community-based nurses is far less direct, mainly accomplished by written orders (not records) and telephone. Such communication is increasingly important as home care has become a growing alternative to nursing home placement and even a substitute for hospital care itself (when, for example, IV antibiotics and enteral feedings can be self-administered). In these circumstances, the American Medical Association and nursing agencies have reminded medical staff of their interprofessional relationships and communications.[117]

The doctor is expected to:

- **Provide complete orders** for patient care goals and treatment
- **Be available** to respond to questions about patient's care, and, if not, to have a substitute, covering colleague, MD or RN
- **Sign and return orders** promptly
- **Advise** on new diagnoses, treatment or referrals
- **Participate** in consideration/resolution of ethical issues in home care
- **Maintain courteous and collegial behavior**

The nurse, in turn, is expected to:

- **Notify family about changes** in patient's physical and
- **Provide periodic summaries** of care at home
- **Discuss changes** regarding medications, limitations, and development of new symptoms

Among these reciprocal duties of exchange, doctors need to be more available to nurses as the latter care for increasingly sick patients at home.

Epilogue

Clearly, optimal care of patients in our increasingly specialized, corporate, complex health care system requires a renewed attention to communication among health care professionals. That renewed attention to doctor-doctor and doctor-nurse relationships is not only for the benefit and needs of patients, but also for the needs of professionals themselves. In today's changing corporate medical world, cooperative collegial relationships maintain the professionalism and morale of the doctor in doctoring, the nurse in nursing, and, in a world where, as Ronald Dworkin notes, the doctor is publicly viewed as a businessman, part-time worker, and body engineer.[118]

These relationship/communication themes may be missing in the classroom training of doctors and nurses — and may not necessarily be "learned on-the-job." More often, even when taught, appropriate doctor-doctor or doctor-nurse communications may not be acted out because self-correcting processes are not in place. While medical schools and hospitals are committed to professional directed care and learning with educational feedback, too often feedback as a neutral and supportive exchange among staff is not practiced — especially when the feedback is over conflicts about process, costs, and specialty jurisdictions of care rather than over knowledge about disease and treatment.

The outcomes and experience of the process of care have importance for the doctor, and certainly for the patient. Better doctor-doctor and doctor-nurse relationships are needed for the improvement of patient care and the professionalism of practitioners. We hope this manual can be used to remind us of the importance of supportive colleague relationships and how to improve them in the shared care of patients.

Appendix

Partners Principles of Patient Care

- We are committed to providing Partners' highest standards of quality, outcomes and service at each of our Partners sites in a timely manner.
- We will measure our success by clinical outcomes, patient satisfaction, professional satisfaction and optimal resource utilization; and we will constantly seek to improve.
- We will affirm that patients have control of their choice of physician and site of care whenever possible, and are provided appropriate and timely information in order to make those decisions.
- We will develop methods and materials to fully inform patients and their families regarding their medical condition and their therapeutic choices.
- We will offer our patients and their families the full array of services provided by Partners physicians and clinical services to facilitate appropriate care.
- We will respect and support the unique relationship of each patient with his or her primary physician (generalist or specialist).
- When the patient is admitted to the hospital, a single physician will assume primary responsibility for the patient's total care and will be available to the patient, family, and the referring physician in fulfilling that role.
- We will work as a team to optimize and coordinate care of patients at the various Partners sites. This process requires clear communication and respecting each other's roles.
- We will seek to use the most effective health care technology and have it available to all our patients.

Acknowledgments

MGH colleagues who have read this manuscript in its many stages with encouragement, suggestions, and comments, or, we surmise, with uncertain endorsements or simply toleration (when we did not hear), are many — a large sample of the staff from general medicine, the medical specialties, nursing and surgery: David Staison, James Richter, David Ratner, Andrew Warshaw, Andrew Billings, Les Fang, Lloyd Axelrod, Gil Daniels, Fred Ackroyd, Kim Eagle, Allan Goroll, John Goodson, Kate Treadway, Alan Friedlich, Isaac Schiff, Gerald Foster, Edwin Maynard, James Dineen, Steven Levisohn, Jerry Younger, Robert Boyd, Jose Vega, Charles McCabe, Alasdair Conn, Michael Barry, William Beck, Barbara Chase, Sharon Follaytar, Roman DeSanctis, Gerald Austen, Hermes Grillo, Stephen Krane, Daniel Federman, Morton Swartz, Edward Ryan, George Baker, Adolph Hutter.

Colleagues outside MGH include: John B. McKinlay (Sociology), Boston University; Stanley Reiser (Ethics-History), University of Texas Medical School; Bertram Bell (Medicine), New York University Medical School; James Pittman (Medicine), University of Alabama Medical School; Frederick Hafferty (Sociology), University of Minnesota Medical School Duluth; Lewis J. Dimsdale (Medicine), Ft. Lauderdale, Florida, Thomas Inui (Medicine), Harvard Community Health Plan.

We are most indebted to Dr. Joan LaRovere, formerly of the College of Physicians and Surgeons, Columbia University, now of Brompton Hospital, London, England, for reference assistance while a medical student, to Catherine Walsh for editorial review, and to Linda Lufkin, Amy Barry, and Sarah Bollinger for manuscript typing/retyping.

References

1. Cabot, R.C. The achievements, standards, and prospects of the Massachusetts General Hospital. Ether Day Address. Boston: Privately printed, Massachusetts General Hospital, 1919.
2. Cabot, R.C. Fee splitting and unnecessary operations. *S Med Surg J* 1929.
3. Stoeckle, J.D. Physicians train and tell. *Harv Med Sch Alum Bull* 1987; 61: 9–11.
4. Shem, S. *The House of God.* New York: Dell, 1978.
5. Komaromg, M., Bindman, A.B., Haber, R.J., Sande, M.A. Sexual harassment in medical training. *N Engl J Med* 1993; 328: 322–326.
6. Rosenberg, D.A., Silver, H.K. Medical student abuse: an unnecessary and preventable cause of stress. *JAMA* 1984; 251: 739–742.
7. Baldwin, De W.C., Daughertry, S.R., Eckengels C.J. Student perceptions of mistreatment and harassment during medical school. A survey often United States schools. *Am J Med* 1991; 155: 140–145.
8. Sheehan, K.H., Sheehan, D.V., White, K., Leibowitz, A., Baldwin, De W.C. Student perceptions of mistreatment and misconduct in medical school. *JAMA* 1990; 263: 533–537.
9. Spiegel, D.A., Smolen, R.C., Jonas, C.K. Interpersonal conflicts involving students in clinical medical education. *J Med Ed* 1985; 60: 819–829.
10. Baldwin, De W.C., Daugherty, S.R., Rowley, B.D. Racial and ethnic discrimination during residency: Results of a National Survey. *Acad Med* 1994; 69: 419–521.
11. Silver, H.K., Glicken, A.D. Medical student abuse, incidence, severity, significance. *JAMA* 1990; 263: 527–532.
12. Friedson, E. *Doctoring Together: A Study of Professional Social Control.* New York: Elsevier Scientific Publishing. 1985.
13. Bosk, C. *Forgive and Remember, Managing Medical Failure.* Chicago: University of Chicago Press, 1977.
14. Good, M.J. *American Medicine, Quest for Competence.* Berkeley: University of California Press, 1995.
15. Stoeckle JD, Ronan LJ, Emaneul LL, Ehrlich CM. A manual on manners and courtesies in the shared care of patients. J Clin Ethics 1997;8:22–33.
16. Verney, R.E. (Ed.). *The Student Life, The Philosophy of Sir William Osler.* Edinburgh: E. and S. Livingstone, 1960.
17. Stoeckle. J.D. *The tasks of care: the humanistic aspects of medical education.* Nourishing the Humanistic in Medicine. (Eds.). Rogers, W.E., Barnard, D. Pittsburgh: University of Pittsburgh Press, 1979.
18. Stoeckle, J.D., Ronan, L., Ehrlich, C., Roberts, D. The uses of shadowing the doctor-and patient: On seeing and hearing the work of care. *J Gen Med* 1993; 8: 561–563.
19. Cushing, H. *The Medical Career.* Boston: Little Brown, 1940.
20. Berczeller, P.H. The malignant consultation syndrome. *Hosp Prac* September 1991; 29–31.
21. McKinlay, J.B., Stoeckle, J.D. Corporatization and the social transformation of medicine. *J Intern Health Serv* 1988; 18: 191–205.
22. Stoeckle, J.D., Reiser, S.J. The corporate organization of hospital work. *Ann Intern Med* 1992; 116: 407–413.
23. Sulmasy, D.P. Physicians, cost control, and ethics. *Ann Intern Med,* 1992; 116: 920–926.
24. Cardiologists provide better care for heart failure patients. *Internal Medicine World Report,* May 1–14, 1996; 26.
25. Greenfield, S., Rogers, W., Mangotich, M., Carney, M.F., Tarlov, A. Outcomes of patients with hypertension and noninsulin dependent diabetes mellitus treated by different systems and specialties. *JAMA* 1995; 274: 1436–1444.
26. Lipsky, P.E., Burnside, J.W. Personal communication on evidence-based algorithm for diagnosis and treatment of joint disorders. University of Texas, Southwestern Medical Center, 1996.
27. Kassier, J.P. The next transformation of health care delivery. *N EngJ Med* 1995; 332: 52–53.

28. Kirk, M.O. The virtual office bumps into some very real limits. *New York Times*, March 8, 1996: 10.
29. Women and Minorities on U.S. Medical School Faculties. Washington: Association of American Medical Colleges, 1988.
30. Schiff, G.D., Goldfield, N. Deming meets Braverman: Towards a progressive analysis of the continuous quality improvement paradigm. *Intl J Health Serv* 1994; 24: 655–673.
31. Best practices and proven strategies for medical managing. Information sharing, idea exchange, help hospitals refine, improve outcomes. *Phys Manager*, 1994; 5: 8.
32. Emmanuel, L.L. Professional response to demands for accountability: practical recommendations regarding ethical aspects of patient care. *Ann Intern Med* 1996; 124: 240–249.
33. Institute of Medicine. *The Computer-based Patient Record: an Essential Technology for Health Care.* Washington: National Academy Press, 1991.
34. Reiser, S.J. The coming resurgence of the generalism in medicine, its technological and conceptual basis. *Pharos* Winter 1995; 8–11.
35. Bruhn, J.G., Levine, H.G., Levine, P.L. *Managing Boundaries in the Health Professions.* Springfield: EC Thomas, 1993.
36. Bhopal, R. Public health medicine and primary health care: convergent, divergent, or parallel paths? *Intl J Epidemiology and Comm Health*, 1995; 49: 113–116.
37. Stoeckle, J.D., Ronan, L. Lower professional incomes could improve care. *Physician's News Digest*, 1994; 8: 5.
38. Present state and future needs of general practice, report from general practice, No. 16. J Royal Col Gen Practitioners 1973; March: 1–59.
39. Stoeckle, J.D. The citadel cannot hold: technologies go outside the hospital, patients and doctors, too. *Milbank Mem Quart* 1995; 73: 31–7.
40. Codman, E.A. *A Study in Hospital Efficiency.* Boston: privately printed, 1916.
41. Hulburt, A. Why manners matter, a review. *The New Republic* December 6, 1982; 24–27.
42. Council of Ethical and Judicial Affairs. Code of Medical Ethics, current opinions with annotations. Chicago: AMA, 1994.
43. Martin, J. *Miss Manners' Guide to Excruciatingly Correct Behavior.* New York: Athenaeum, 1982.
44. Percival, T. *Medical Ethics or a Code of Institutes and Precepts* (reprinted). Birmingham: Classics in Medical Literature, 1803 and 1987.
45. Nutting, P.A., Franks, P., Clancy, C.M. Referral and consultation in primary care: Do we understand what we're doing? *J Fam Practitioners*, 1992; 35: 21–23.
46. Hines, R.M., Curry, D.J. The consultation process and physician satisfactions review of referral patterns in three urban family practice units. *Can Med Assoc J* 1978; 118: 1065–1073.
47. Ludke, R.L. An examination of the factors that influence patient referral decisions. *Med Care* 1982; 20: 782–796.
48. Williams, P.T., Peet, G. Difference in the value of clinical information: referring physicians versus consulting specialists. *J Am Board Fam Practitioners* 1994; 7: 292–302.
49. McPhee, S.J., Lo, B., Saika, G.Y., Moltier, R. How good is communication between primary care physicians and subspecialty consultants? *Arch Intern Med* 1984; 144: 1265–1269.
50. Hansen, J.P., Brown, S.E., Sullivan, R.J., Muhlbaier, L.H. Factors related an effective referral and consultative process. *J Fam Practitioners* 1982; 15: 651–650.
51. Epstein, R.M. Communication between primary care physician and consultants. *Arch Fam Med* 1995; 4: 403–409.
52. Lee, T., Pappius, E.M., Goldman, L. Impact of inter-physician communication on effectiveness of medical consultations. *Am J Med* 1983; 74: 106–112.
53. Cummins, R.D., Smith, R.W., Inui, T.S. Communication failure in primary care, failure of consultants to provide follow-up information. *JAMA* 1980; 243: 1650–1652.
54. Hennen, B.K.E. Family doctors consult with specialists for non-medical reasons. *Can Med Assoc J* 1992; 147; 609–610.

55. Armstrong, D., Fry, J., Armstrong, P. Doctor's perceptions of pressures from patients for referral. *Brit Med J* 1991; 302: 1186–1188.
56. Emmanuel. L., Richter, J. The consultant and the physician-patient relationship. *Arch Intern Med* 1994; 54: 1785–1790.
57. Cabot, R.C. *The Training of the Physician.* Boston: JB Lippincott, 1916.
58. *Counsels and Ideas and Selected Aphorisms from the Writings of William Osler.* Birminigham: Classics in Medical Literature, 1985.
59. Barlow, D.T.C. *British General Practice, a Personal Study for Students.* London: HK Lewis Ltd., 1973.
60. Lipsitt, D.R. The doctor as patient. *Psychological Opinion* 1975; 12: 20–25.
61. Levy, M.A, Arnold, R.M., Fine, A.J., Kapook, W.N. Professional courtesy — current practices and attitudes. *N EngJ Med* 1993; 329: 1627–1631.
62. Shanafelt, T.D., Bradley, K.A., Wipf, J.E., Back A.L. Burnout and self-reported patient care in an Internal Medicine Residency Program. *Ann of Int Med* 2002; 136: 358–367.
63. Meier, D.E., Back, A.L., Morrison, R.S. The inner life of physicians and case of the seriously ill. *JAMA 2001*; 286: 2007–2014
64. Spiro, H.A. When doctors get sick. *Persp Bio Med* 1987; 31: 117–33.
65. Marzuk, P.M. When the patient is a physician. *N EngJ Med* 1987; 317: 1409–33.
66. Duffy, J.C., Litin, E.A. *The Physician-Patient: The Emotional Health of Physicians.* Springfield: Thomas, 35–41, 1967.
67. *Through the Patient's Eyes, Understanding and Promoting Patient-centered Care.* (Eds.). Gerther, M., Edgman-Levitan, S., Daley, J., Delbanco, T.L. San Francisco: Jossey-Bass, 1993.
68. Lazarus, A. From stethoscope to spread sheet: The physician with the MBA. *Pharos* Spring 1995; 20–23.
69. Hafferty, F.W., Light, D.W. Professional dynamics and the changing nature of medical work. *J Health and Soc Beh*, extra issue 1995; 132–153.
70. Harrison, S., Pollitt, C. *Controlling Health Professionals, the Future of Work and the Organization in the National Health Service.* Philadelphia: Open University Press, 1994.
71. Stoeckle, J.D. Working on the factory floor. *Ann Intern Med* 1987; 107: 250–251.
72. Compensation and management trends. *Physician Manager* 1996; 7: 6.
73. Lombardi, D.N. *Thriving in an Age of Changes: Practical Strategies For Health Care Leaders.* Chicago: Am College Health Care Executives, 1996.
74. Leander, W.J. *Patient First: Experience of a Patient-Centered Pioneer.* Chicago: Health Administration Press, 1996.
75. Kletke, P.R., Emmons, D.W., Gillis, K.D. Current trends in physician practice arrangements, from owners to employees. *JAMA* 1996; 276: 555–560.
76. Allsop, J., Mulcahy, L. *Regulating Medical Work: Formal and Informal Controls.* Philadelphia: Open University Press, 1996.
77. Wachter, R.M., Goldman, L. The emerging role of "hospitalists" in the American health system. *N EngJ Med* 1996; 335: 514–517.
78. Lee, D. Firms — a growing delivery model. *Soc Gen Intern Med Forum* 1996; 19: 1: 6.
79. Puma, J.L. House physicians, accountability and responsibilities. *Arch Intern Med* 1996; 156: 2529–2533.
80. Wachter, R.M., Goldman, Lee. The hospital movement 5 years later. *JAMA* 202; 287: 487–494
81. Cabot, R.C. The effect of doctoring on the doctor. *The World Tomorrow*, February 1922; 43–44.
82. Berwick, D. Not again! Preventing errors lies in redesign — not exhortation. *Brit Med J — USA* 2001; 1: 155–6.
83. Leape, L.L. Errors in medicine. *JAMA*, 1994; 272: 1851–1857.
84. Blumenthal, D. Making medical errors with "medical treasures." *JAMA* 1994; 272: 1867–1868.
85. Lazare, A. Shame, humiliation and stigma in the medical encounter. *Arch Intern Med* 1987; 147: 1653–1658.

86. Christenson, J.F., Levinson, W., Dunn, P.M. The heart of darkness: The impact of perceived mistakes on physicians. *J Gen Intern Med* 1992; 7: 424–431.
87. Pekkanen, J. *Doctors Talk about Themselves.* New York: Delacorte Press, 1988.
88. *Doctor to Doctor Writing and Talking about Patients,* a collection of essays from a Nuffield Working Party on Communication. (Eds.). Walton, S.J., McLaughlin, G., London: Nuffield Provincial Hospital Trust, 1984.
89. *Taking Care of Doctors,* reducing avoidable stress and improving services for doctors who fall ill. London: Nuffield Provincial Hospitals Trust, 1996.
90. McKevitt, C., Morgan, M., Simpson, J., Holland, W. *Doctor's Health and the Needs for Services.* London: Nuffield Provincial Hospitals Trust, 1996.
91. Gutman, E.J., Salzman, G.A. Much ado about nothing. *Modern Pathology* 1999; 12: 95–97.
92. Stern, D.T., Caldicott, C.V. Turfing, patients in the balance. *J Gen Intern Med* 1999: 14: 243–248.
93. Regulations for Residents and House Officers. Massachusetts General Hospital. Privately published, author unacknowledged, but written by Dr. Charles Short, the hospital's first chief resident, 1931.
94. *New Pathways to Medical Education, Learning to Learn at Harvard Medical School.* (Eds). Tosteson, D.C., Adelstein, S.J., Carver, S.T. Cambridge: Harvard University Press, 1994.
95. Cassell, E.J. Practice versus theory in academic medicine: the conflict between house officers and attending physicians. *Bull NY Acad Med* 1984; 60: 297–308.
96. Council Report. Disputes between medical supervisors and trainees. *JAMA* 1994; 272: 1861–1865.
97. Wartman, S.A. Managed care and its effect on residency training in internal medicine. *Arch Intern Med* 1993; 154: 2539–2544.
98. A Synopsis of the New Medicare Rules on Payment for Teaching Physicians. Washington: Association of American Medical Colleges, 1996.
99. Scannell, J.G. Let us now praise famous men. *Am J Surgeons* 1974; 127: 365–370.
100. Yedidia, M.J., Lipkin, M., Schwartz, M.D., Hirschkorn, C. Doctors as workers: work-hour regulation and intern's reception of responsibility, quality of care, and training. *J Gen Intern Med* 1993; 8: 429–435.
101. Editorial. Burnished or burned out: the delights and dangers of working in health. *Lancet* 1994; 344: 1583.
102. Bell BM. Supervision, not regulation of hours, is the key to improving the quality of patient care. *JAMA* 1993; 269: 403–404.
103. Messner, E. *Resilience Enhancement for the Resident Physician.* Durant, O.K.: Essential Medical Information Systems, 1993.
104. Balint M. The Doctor, his Patient, and the Illness. London: Pitman Books, 1964.
105. Reiser, S.J. *Science, Pedagogy and the Transformation of Empathy in Medicine,* Chapter 12, Empathy and the Practice of Medicine (Eds.). Spiro, H., McCrea, M., Cureieu, M.G., Peschel, E., and St. James, D. New Haven: Yale University Press, 1993.
106. Branch, W., Pels, R.J., Lawrence, R.S., Arky, R. Becoming a doctor, critical-incident reports from third-year medical students. *N EngJ Med* 1993; 329: 1130–1132.
107. Martin, J. *Common Courtesy.* Pleasantville, NY: Akadine Press, 1996.
108. Knowles, J.H. *The Teaching Hospital in Hospitals, Doctors, and the Public Interest.* (Ed.). Knowles, J. H. Cambridge: Harvard University Press, 1965.
109. Fagin, C.M. Collaboration between nurse and physician no longer a choice. *Acad Med* 1992; 67: 295–303.
110. Stein, L.I. The doctor-nurse game. *Arch Gen Psychiatry,* 1967; 6: 699–703.
111. Stein, L.I., Watts, D.T., Howell, T. The doctor-nurse game revisited. *N Engl J Med* 1990; 322: 546–549.
112. Makadon, H.J., Gibbons, T. Nurses and physicians: prospects for collaboration. *Ann Intern Med* 1985; 103: 134–135.

113. Georgopoulos, B.S. Organizational structure and the performance of hospital emergency services. *Ann Emer Med* 1985; 14, 677–684.
114. DeFede, J.P., Dhanens, B.E., Keltner, N.L. Cost benefits of patient-controlled analgesia. *Nurse Manager* 1989; 20: 34–35.
115. Knaus, W.A., Draper, E.A., Wagner, D.P., Zimmerman, J.E. An evaluation of outcome from intensive care in major medical centers. *Ann Intern Med* 1986; 104: 410–418.
116. Leape, L.L. Systems analysis of adverse drug events. *JAMA* 1995; 274: 35–43.
117. Recommendations and regulations. (1) All Care Visiting Nurse Association of Greater Lynn, (2) Malden Visiting Nurse Association, Malden MA and (3) Special Care Home Health Service, Wilmington, MA on "Mutual Responsibility Guidelines for Collaborative Care," 1995.
118. Dworkin, R.W. Why Doctors are Down. *Commentary* May 2001; 43–47.